All About Bone

An Owner's Manual

Irwin M. Siegel, M.D.

Demos Medical Publishing, Inc., 386 Park Avenue South,
New York, New York 10016

Library of Congress Cataloging-in-Publication Data

Siegel, Irwin M., 1927–
    All about bone : an owner's manual / Irwin M. Siegel.
      p. cm.
    Includes index.
    ISBN 1–888799–16–1
    1. Bones—Diseases—Popular works. 2. Musculoskeletal system—
—Diseases—Popular works. 3. Orthopedics—Popular works.
I. Title.
RC930.S47 1998
616.7′1—dc21

                    98-9675
                    CIP

Made in the United States of America

This book
is for my students,
who have kept me boning up
to meet the challenge of their
searching minds. No bones about it.
They have taught me much.

In Appreciation

I would really be a bonehead if I did not thank the following people for their help with this book:

Mrs. Alice Thanner for her proficient secretarial services.

Mrs. Jackie Abern for expert typing and proofreading the manuscript.

Ms. Iris Sachs for bibliographic assistance.

Artist Kurt Peterson for his outstanding illustrations.

My wife, Barbara, for accepting with understanding the evenings apart and the homebound weekends while I isolated myself to work and rework the book.

Demos Medical Publishing of New York City, and particularly Dr. Diana M. Schneider and Joan Wolk, for patiently and skillfully shepherding the book through editing and publication.

My colleagues, Dr. Levon Toupouzian and the late Robert Keagy, for reviewing the manuscript and offering helpful criticism.

I would truly have been "out on a limb" without those listed, as well as the many colleagues and friends whose encouragement brought *All About Bone* to completion.

Preface

Bone is one of the most interesting and unique tissues of the human body. I have been studying bone for more than 40 years, and I am still impressed by the wonder of nature's handiwork expressed in this unusual material.

I decided to write this book in response to the many questions patients have asked me about bone during the course of my orthopaedic practice. Some of them wanted to know about a specific disease of bone or joint, like osteoporosis or arthritis. Others asked about injuries, such as fractures or sprains. Still others were curious about how bones metabolized, grew, or mended. So I decided to write a book "all about bone" for anyone who is interested in how this important part of the body functions, both in health and in disease.

Although I have tried to include what the average reader might want to know about bone, *All About Bone* is far from "everything about bone." So if it does not answer your questions, I encourage you to ask your doctor. And, of course, consult a physician for any health problem, because this book is not intended to provide instruction for individual diagnosis or treatment. No single book or any one person has all the answers. But it is, after all, your body, you are the owner, and you should keep picking a bone with anyone you have to until you are satisfied with the answers you get. I sincerely hope you find *All About*

Bone informative, and I also hope you enjoy reading the book as much as I enjoyed writing it.

Irwin M. Siegel, M.D.
Evanston, Illinois

Introduction

A SKELETAL HISTORICAL PERSPECTIVE

"And the Lord God caused a deep sleep to fall upon the man, and he slept; and he took one of his ribs, and closed up the place with flesh instead thereof, and the rib, which the Lord God had taken from the man, made He a woman, and brought her unto the man." Thus, in the Book of Genesis, Chapter II, Lines 21–23, the first of many references to bone is made in the Old Testament. "This is now bone of my bones. . ." said the man, and thereafter, a blood relative was referred to as "my own bone and flesh." The biblical term for bone, *etzem,* is derived from the Hebrew, *otzem,* meaning to press together, thus hard, essence. Figuratively, it is used to denote strength. The bone of Luz was regarded as the source of life and yes, indeed, the focus of resurrection. This bone was said to be located near the sacrum (a bony structure at the base of the spine, so named because it was regarded as sacred).

The oldest diseases known to man have engraved their history of destruction on bone. Archaeological digs have unearthed evidence of arthritis, syphilis, tuberculosis, and other degenerative diseases that affect bone. Attempts at treating disease through primitive operations on bone also have been found. Demonstration of trephination (opening holes in the skull) has been discovered in widely scattered locales, but mostly in France, some ten thousand years B.C., and South America, at least several centuries before Columbus discovered the New World.

The Edwin Smith papyrus, of Egyptian origin and composed circa 1650 B.C., is among the earliest known medical writings. It describes how to diagnose and treat 48 injuries to bones and joints. Bones have been manipulated for ritual and aesthetic reasons from skull molding in primitive tribes to foot binding in ancient China.

Hippocrates (circa 400 B.C.), the greatest of the Greek physicians, wrote extensively on broken bones and dislocated joints. He treated fractures with clay or starch casts and dislocations with the help of a bench (Hippocratic scamnum) fitted to hold the patient and apply those forces needed to reduce the dislocated joint. An ironic historical twist is that medieval inquisitors later used the scamnum, devised for healing, as the rack for torture.

Renaissance artists, particularly Leonardo DaVinci, studied the skeleton in detail and drew it accurately. Leonardo compared the bones to architectural supports and the joints to systems of levers. The armorers of the Middle Ages were the first prosthetists (limb makers), applying their craft to the fashioning of limbs to replace those lost to the blades and musketry of ancient warfare.

Toward the end of the seventeenth century, bone began to be scientifically studied through the aid of newly developed instrumentation, such as the microscope. The medical-surgical specialty that treats diseases and conditions of the bones and joints was first codified by the Paris professor of medicine Nicholas Andre (1658–1741). He named this branch of medicine *orthopaedics,* from the Greek: *orthos* (straight) and *paidios* (child), and elaborated a system of splinting and exercise to prevent and treat postural deformities.

Many other physicians turned their attention to the investigation of bone. Among these was the great English surgeon scientist John Hunter (1728–1793). His many discoveries included the observation that bone was living tissue that changed its metabolism and form in response to life's stresses and strains. The discovery of x-ray by William Roentgen in 1895 opened a new era in the study of bone. For the first time, bones could be seen without invading the living body. Roentgen was awarded the first Nobel Prize in physics in 1901 for his monumental work.

There are 206 bones in the human body. Each arm has 32 bones, each leg has 31, the axial skeleton has 80, of which 29 are in the skull, 26 in the spine, and 25 in the chest. They form numerous joints and are heir to more than 500 diseases. Our skeleton not only furnishes support and protection for our vital organs, but also provides a protective site for the blood-forming system (bone marrow) and a reservoir for minerals, particularly calcium and phosphate.

Through its structural support for the mechanical action of muscles, the skeleton permits us to defy the forces of gravity in standing upright and to move in not only functional but also sometimes exquisite and amazing ways.

Compact bone has a tensile strength as high as 20,000 pounds and an average compressive strength of 30,000 pounds per square inch, the same as aluminum or soft steel. However, bone has an advantage in that it is considerably lighter and exhibits a greater elasticity than either of these metals (bone is about as elastic as spruce), which is important to the skeleton's ability to withstand impact. All the while it is metabolically active, renewing itself completely in less than seven years. Of the tissues of the body, bone is unique in mending itself not with scar tissue but with new bone tissue.

This book will tell you about the structure and nature of bone. It will inform you about skeletal injuries and diseases of bone. It will teach you how to keep your bones and joints healthy and functioning at top form. It will review such subjects as exercise, back and neck care, athletic injuries, foot care, fractures, posture, and much more. We will survey the skeletal system from the top of the skull to the tips of the toes, and review its functions in health and its treatment in disease. This book is *All About Bone*.

Contents

1

Consider Bone

Bone of my bone, and flesh of my flesh.

Genesis I, 28

The unique tissue that is bone is found only in vertebrates—animals with backbones. A rigid skeleton would be a distinct disadvantage for water-dwelling animals. As land-roaming vertebrates developed, they began to use bone for support, to protect their internal organs, as a base for muscular attachment, and for the leverage necessary to assist in pulling. Sea mammals, such as the walrus and its cousin the sea lion, have put bone to uncommon use by sporting rigid penile bones. This is known as the os penis or baculum. In fact, all carnivores (dogs, cats, seals, bears), rodents, bats, insectivores, and primates (except man) have one, considering it may be variously shaped and made of cartilage as well as bone. Whales, most marsupials, and the hoofed mammals are not so blessed. Bone also serves the important function of regulating internal chemistry through calcium and phosphorus exchange. We are going to examine this wonderful material that forms the framework of the human body.

Newborn infants have approximately 350 individual bones. By fusion and rearrangement during growth, they develop into their adult counterparts. The adult skeleton (Greek: *skeletos*, meaning dried up) usually contains 206 bones, although some people are born with either an extra pair of ribs or one pair less (most commonly in Mongols). It was once believed that men had

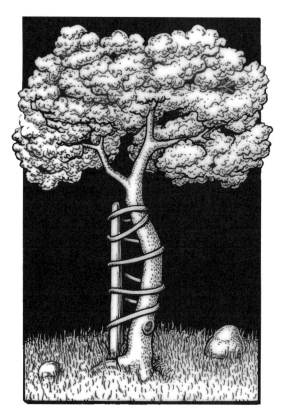

FIGURE 1-1   The splinted tree emblem of Nicolas Andry (1658–1742), who published the first book on orthopaedics in 1741.

one less rib than women because of the description in Genesis of the creation of Eve from one of Adam's ribs. Someone finally counted and compared a man's rib cage with that of a woman, putting this myth to rest.

STRUCTURE

Bone consists of living cells held in a hard intercellular material. This material is composed of collagen, a fibrous protein similar in structure and organization to ligaments, tendons, and skin. This collagenous matrix is mineralized, mainly with calcium and phosphorus. The intimate blending of the hard and resilient components in bone makes it almost equally resistant to compression and tension. This is in contrast to most of the

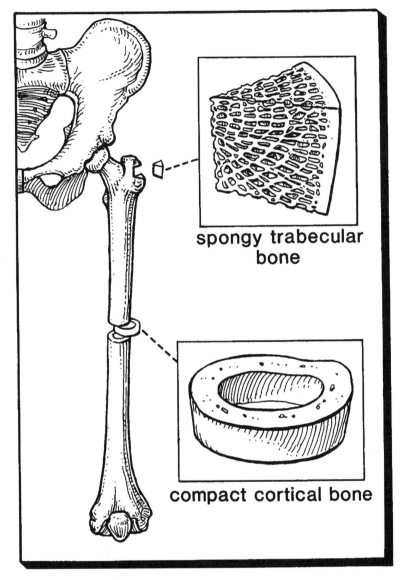

spongy trabecular
bone

compact cortical bone

FIGURE 1-2   Bone Architecture

structural materials that we commonly use, which are usually better in one respect than another. The two-phased materials used in bone give it hardness, rigidity, *and* flexibility. This is similar to other two-phased materials, such as fiberglass or bamboo. Because an element of viscous flow is present, bone is stiffer during rapid deformation than during slow deformation.

A variety of features adapt bone to its specific functions within the body. A tubular structure, typical of the shafts of many long limb bones (and tubular furniture as well), is the strongest yet lightest arrangement that can be designed. In such long limb bones, the thickness of the shell (compact cortical bone) is greatest at the midshaft, where torsion and bending stresses are greatest. Bony *trabeculae* (Latin, meaning little beams) are strengthening girders of spongy cancellous bone within the bones that support the mechanical stresses involved in walking, running, and jumping. These trabeculae provide maximum strength where bones articulate as joints. Here, surprisingly large compression forces may be generated. For instance, in standing the hip takes half the body weight, and the pull of stabilizing muscles (muscle moments) may multiply this sixfold. Obviously, the full body weight is carried alternatively by each hip when one is running or walking. An average adult man bears a hip load of 600 pounds with each step, and this can easily be doubled during powerful exertion.

Bone appears to be one of the strongest materials devised by nature. One cubic inch of bone can withstand loads of up to 20,000 pounds, well over four times the strength of concrete. This is all the more remarkable when one considers that bone accounts for only 14 percent of total body weight, or approximately 20 to 25 pounds. Its strength is derived by weaving protein and mineral into a resilient bony fabric. Almost two-thirds of bone consists of various minerals, mainly complex calcium and phosphorus compounds containing traces of sodium, zinc, lead, and other elements. The crystalline structure formed by these salts lends bone its hardness and rigidity. Why calcium? As Loren Eisely said in *The Immense Journey,* "Only because of its history. Elements more numerous than calcium in the Earth's crust could have been used to build the skeleton. Our history is the reason—we came from the water. It was there that cells took the lime habit, and they kept it after we came ashore." Deer antlers are bony outgrowths on a base of keratin (the protein that forms fingernails). They are the only bones that are shed each year. Other animal horn, including that of the rhinoceros (which is sought for its aphrodisiac quality), is keratin on a bony core. Ivory tusks are modified tooth dentin.

The remaining portion of bone is composed of collagen, the elastic protein that makes glue when bones are boiled. Fibers of collagen studded with crystals wind themselves around each other like strands of rope fibers. Remove the mineral in bone—this can be done by placing a chicken bone in vinegar (acetic acid) for a few days—and the bone becomes so pliable that it can be tied in a knot.

The skeleton demonstrates the use of state-of-the-art engineering principles to provide the greatest strength with the least material. It closely resembles coral in structure, and like such meshworks it is both sturdy and delicate. The femur, or thigh bone, is the longest and strongest of all human bones. It may be called on to resist a compressive force of more than 1,000 pounds per cubic inch during walking. What is even more remarkable is that, unlike nonliving materials such as concrete or steel, bone remodels itself under stress. It does this through a complex system of cellular communication that is electrical in nature. For example, cavalrymen were known to "acquire" new bone in their buttocks and thighs in response to the muscular tensions that occur with constant riding.

Like any well-recognized factory, bone divides labor between its four major types of cells. *Osteoblasts* make bone, *osteoclasts* remodel bone, *osteocytes* govern its metabolism, and a group of uncharacterized basic structures termed *undifferentiated mesenchymal cells* stand ready to evolve into -blasts, -clasts, or -cytes if and when needed. With the exception of dental enamel, bone is the hardest tissue in the body. Now let's see how bone renews itself.

REMODELING, GROWTH, AND DEVELOPMENT

As in any other mammal, human bones are "preformed" in cartilage. This soft tissue model is gradually converted into bone tissue by a bony change called *osteogenesis*. A skeletal outline can be seen in the human embryo at approximately the fifth week of pregnancy. Ossification of bone continues until almost 25 years of age, at which time the cartilage is completely replaced by bone, ending further transformation. A few of the bones of our bodies are not preformed in cartilage. These "membrane bones" form in condensed fibrous tissue. They include the brane bones" form in condensed fibrous tissue. They include the bones of the skull and the clavicle (collarbone).

Long bones grow at each end through a growth plate, or *physis,* as well as from a thin membrane called the *periosteum,* which surrounds the shaft of the bone. Cells from this layer begin to form bone around the middle of a cartilage shaft and continue this process during growth, which allows the bone to increase in diameter as well as in length. At the ends of bones, cartilage cells are destroyed and replaced by bone tissue. These newly deposited cells push the growth plate farther from the center of the shaft until the body has attained its full height, which occurs at approximately 18 years in men and two years earlier in women. During our lifetime, we actually have three skeletons—the first one is made of cartilage, the second of an immature fibrous type bone, and the third of adult bone.

Numerous metabolic influences affect bone growth. Essential monitoring and manufacturing roles in the development of the bony skeleton are played by the availability of minerals such as phosphorus and calcium, vitamins A, D, and C, as well as by the secretions of many endocrine glands, including the thyroid, parathyroid, pituitary, adrenals, and gonads.

The tissues of the body constantly renew themselves. This process is so rapid and so continuous that you hardly have any single cell in your body that you had three years ago. Renewal in soft tissues occurs largely at a molecular level. Bony change occurs by replacing tissue; it is somewhat like urban renewal in that removal of the old bone by resorption must precede new bone deposition. Remodeling is greatest during growth and declines until approximately age 35. After the age of 35, remodeling remains essentially unchanged. After the fourth decade of life, resorption of bone is greater than formation, and a loss of 5 percent to 10 percent of bone mass occurs with each passing decade. This works out to a loss of approximately 4 grams of calcium from the skeleton each year.

The processes of remodeling, growth, and development are under the control of the cells of bone. Osteoclasts secrete enzymes that dissolve bone, and osteoblasts elaborate a protein-like substance, called *osteoid,* which is then mineralized. It is thought that osteocytes, the mainstay cell of mature bone, are also metabolically active and can resorb and even re-form bone on demand.

To keep the delicate mineral chemistry of the body in balance, bone acts as the body's major storehouse for minerals. Approximately half of bone's volume and up to 75 percent of its weight consists of deposited minerals. Almost 90 percent of the calcium and phosphorus in the body is found in the bones. If spread out, the crystal surface exposed to the body fluids in the walls of the skeletal system of an average man would cover 1,500 to 5,000 square meters. This is approximately the size of a football field and provides an enormous surface area across which chemical exchanges of minerals can occur.

Julius Wolff, who was a professor of orthopaedics in Berlin, formulated his famous law of bone modeling late in the nineteenth century. Wolff's law holds that the physical stresses placed on bone initiate accommodative changes in its structure and form. It would seem that small electrical currents are generated from pressure in bone, and these charges stimulate resorption or production in response to the stress imposed.

The human skeleton not only serves to store minerals but also acts as the reservoir that controls the equilibrium of calcium and phosphate in the blood stream. These elements are vital for cardiac function, muscle contractility, cell membrane integrity and permeability, neuromuscular function, and blood clotting. Bone governs the body concentration of calcium and phosphorus through hormonal regulation by parathyroid hormone and calcitonin. This is controlled through "feedback loops" that hormonally link the excretion of calcium and phosphorus by the kidney with the absorption of these ions by the intestine. Vitamin D is required in this metabolic scheme. Calcitonin is a body chemical that inhibits bone resorption. Renovation of bone depends on two of these control loops with negative feedback. Remodeling under Wolff's law may be related to the "piezoelectric properties" of bone crystals, which involve the generation of electricity by crystalline structures under stress. Tension on a bone sets up a negative electrical pole (anode), whereas compression sets up a positive pole (cathode). This process also plays an important role in bone healing.

A number of hormones also play significant roles in the regulation of bone growth and metabolism. These include estrogens, testosterone, thyroid hormone, adrenal gland hormones, insulin, and growth hormone.

It should be obvious that a diet rich in protein and adequate in minerals is necessary for proper bone growth and development. Approximately 1 to 2 grams of calcium per day is advised for adolescents and for pregnant and lactating women. Adults require somewhat less, and postmenopausal women need a little more. The daily recommended allowance for phosphorus is the same as for calcium. Deficiency in these elements results in mineral-poor bone, causing rickets in children and osteomalacia in adults. We discuss this more in the next chapter on osteoporosis. The skeleton also stores magnesium, sodium, and fluoride. Bone can also pick up radium. Once in bone tissue, this element radiates other tissues with its beta particles, causing cancer mutations. The numbers on the faces of clocks used to be coated with radium-impregnated paint to make them glow in the dark. Workers painting these clock dials would point the tip of the paint brush with their lips. Many subsequently died of radium-induced bone cancer.

Vitamins are also essential to the integrity of bone.

❑ Vitamin A is necessary for the proliferation of cartilage and the growth of bone. Too little vitamin A results in poor remodeling, and too much results in thinning and fracture. Eskimos have learned to avoid vitamin A intoxication by not eating the livers of the polar bear or seal, in which vitamin A is highly concentrated.

❑ We need vitamin C for the formation of collagen, and its lack causes scurvy. English sailors were called "limeys" because they were required to suck limes, which are high in vitamin C, to avoid getting scurvy on long sea voyages when other vitamin C–containing food was limited.

❑ Vitamin D is important for the intestinal absorption of calcium, in the regulation of mineral metabolism by the kidney, and for the integrity of bone cells. Rickets due to vitamin D deficiency secondary to lack of adequate exposure to sunshine has been held by some to be the first disease caused by industrial pollution, because it occurred endemically in the smoke-filled, foggy coal mining villages of England and Wales.

Hollow bones are filled with marrow. The ribs, vertebrae, pelvic bones, and skull bones contain red marrow, which produces both red and white blood cells as well as platelets. Long bones are filled with yellow marrow, which consists mostly of fat that serves as a reservoir for energy when other body fat stores are depleted. In anemia, yellow marrow can be converted to red marrow for the manufacture of red blood cells. Traditionally, bone diseases and injuries fall within the purview of orthopaedic surgeons. However, bone problems are often associated with diseases treated by other medical specialists, notably neurologists, rheumatologists, pediatricians, and physiatrists (specialists in physical medicine and rehabilitation). By far, the most common bone disorder is fracture (broken bone). However, physical injury to bone cannot be separated from other conditions. For instance, fracture in a joint can lead to arthritis of that joint (traumatic arthritis), and the presence of osteoporosis (thin bones) predisposes one to fracture.

In children bone problems related to growth and development predominate. An occasional glimpse of a straight and slender female ankle was all that was permitted in proper Victorian England. Nonetheless, this anatomic configuration attested to the fact that the girl did not have bowlegs, a common result of childhood rickets. In young adults traumatic and athletic injuries are frequent; and in the older individual metabolic abnormalities, degenerative diseases, and conditions secondary to deficient circulation predominate.

Bone was initially regarded as a static tissue, and diseases and injuries of bone were looked upon as being strictly mechanical. As an understanding of the metabolic function of bone improved, it was realized that conditions of bone, including fractures, were dynamic in nature. This understanding of the chemical and mechanical function of bone has enabled a more integrated biologic view of bone diseases and injuries.

This chapter has given you a brief overview, a skeleton if you will, of the basic science you need to better grasp the practical advice that the rest of the book provides. With some understanding of what keeps bone strong, the next chapter looks at what occurs when it becomes weak and how we can prevent that from happening.

QUESTIONS AND ANSWERS ABOUT BONE

Q: What determines how much bone we have?

A: Our bone mass is influenced by heredity, nutrition, work, exercise, and hormones. After growth stops, bone mass increases until approximately age 35.

Q: Why don't other tissues calcify like bone does?

A: Although all connective tissues contain bundles of collagen fibers, only bone calcifies. The cells that form the fibers of other connective tissues do not produce enzymes that alter protein so that it will trap calcium. This process is unique to the osteoblast cell, which allows calcification of new bone using calcium in the extracellular fluid, which does not tend to precipitate elsewhere. Also, the principal mineral of bone is a compound of calcium and phosphate called hydroxyapatite. This does not form except under the special conditions that are present in bone, except in part in turkeys, whose tendons often calcify.

Q: How does exercise affect the skeleton?

A: It probably has something to do with the electrical fields produced when bone is under pressure or tension. These electrical fields keep the formation and destruction of bone remodeling in balance. You cannot have strong bone without exercise. While in a state of zero gravity, astronauts must exercise vigorously to minimize loss of mineral from their bones. For long periods in space, when nothing is pressing down on the bones, even vigorous exercise may not suffice to compensate for demineralization. In one study, researchers found a 100 percent increase in the amount of calcium in the urine of the *Skylab* astronauts. This amounts to an overall bone loss of almost one-half a percent a month.

Q: Why do some people need more calcium than others do?

A: Calcium absorption from the diet is inefficient. Mature adults absorb only one-third the calcium from a typical diet. This fraction decreases with age. After menopause it is only one-fourth of oral calcium intake. After calcium is incorporated into the skeleton, some people absorb it better than other people do. There are also some individual differences in calcium elimination. Some people eliminate calcium easily and they need to consume more, sometimes a lot more.

Q: Does anorexia nervosa affect calcium metabolism?

A: Yes, indeed. Young women with anorexia nervosa may develop severe osteoporosis. With inadequate nutritional intake, the body may shut down the production of female hormones, and such patients lose bone just like postmenopausal women do. Dental problems, including periodontal disease, can also result from low calcium intake.

2

Osteoporosis

Thy bones are hollow.

William Shakespeare, Measure for Measure, I,ii,56

Osteoporosis (from the Greek: *osteon,* meaning bone; *poros,* meaning passage; in other words an enlargement of the spaces in bone or porous bone) is a disorder of bone metabolism that causes a loss of mass in the skeleton, with subsequent weakening of bone. It is the most common skeletal malady. Only arthritis causes more disability in the elderly.

Osteoporosis is more prevalent in women than in men. Approximately 25 million Americans have some form of the disorder, and 80 percent of them are women. This is the "weak bones" condition that many women develop after menopause.

Osteoporosis leaves the bones thin and fragile. Because of this, they break easily; most fractures in women over the age of 50 and most of the hip fractures that occur in the United States are secondary to osteoporosis. It costs approximately $10 billion dollars each year to treat patients who have osteoporosis, mostly for the care of fractures.

Osteoporosis is to some extent preventable. There are things you can do throughout life to prevent osteoporosis, and if you already have this condition, there are ways you can live with it in comfort and safety.

Almost one of every four women over the age of 65 develops a broken bone secondary to osteoporosis. These fractures are usually of a vertebra (backbone), neck of the femur (hip), wrist, or rib. Such a break may result from minimal trauma because of the thinness of the bone involved. The fractures are usually very painful.

The National Osteoporosis Foundation claims that osteoporosis "has been under-diagnosed, under-reported, and inadequately researched in men." American men over the age of 50 stand a greater chance of suffering an osteoporosis-related fracture than of developing clinical prostate cancer. One of eight such men will break a bone as a result of osteoporosis. A total of 100,000 men a year break their hips. One-third of them die within a year because of complications related to the fracture, the surgery to repair the break, or bed confinement.

The incidence of osteoporosis in men is expected to rise as more men live into their seventies and beyond. In a study of more than 800 Australian men, those in their late seventies had three times as many fractures as those in their early sixties, and men in their eighties had seven times as many fractures as did men in their sixties. Women lose bone much more quickly than men of the same age during the 10 years immediately after the onset of menopause. By age 65 or 70, however, men and women lose bone mass at the same rate. Calcium absorption decreases in both sexes with advancing age.

This chapter is an overview of osteoporosis and looks at those factors that have been associated with increased risk for this disease. I discuss methods for early detection of osteoporosis, ways to prevent the condition, risk factors, suggestions for living with osteoporosis, and state-of-the-art methods of treating it.

CAUSES

As you learned in Chapter 1, bone is a "bank" for calcium and other essential minerals. Osteoporosis results in a loss of bone mineral density and appears as a diffuse thinning of bone on an x-ray film. There is increased porosity of the cancellous (spongy trabecular) bone and a decrease in the thickness of cortical (compact) bone.

In the healthy individual there is a constant movement of calcium and other minerals in and out of the skeleton, accompanied by a continual remodeling of the bones through a lifelong process of deposition and resorption. Osteoporosis occurs when the balance of these processes tilts toward resorption. As we learned in Chapter 1, deposition usually dominates resorption until approximately age 35, after which bone mass begins to decrease. This normal decrease may in time lead to osteoporosis. In women hormones play a significant role in this process, because estrogen appears to directly affect bone-resorbing cells (osteoclasts). Consequently, there is an accelerated loss of bone in postmenopausal women, or in any woman who has oligomenorrhea (infrequent or scant periods), long menstrual cycles, amenorrhea (absence of menses), or three to six missed cycles, or those who have had a surgically induced menopause. Female athletes afflicted with stress fractures may be expressing premature osteoporosis as a result of the cycle abnormalities they frequently experience.

Other factors also play a role. Those who have a family history of osteoporosis seem to be more prone to the disease. Women who are thin and petite, of white or Asian ancestry, or who have thin, fair skin are also more likely to have osteoporosis. Other factors that have a negative effect on bone include physical inactivity, a history of nontraumatic fracture, alcohol consumption (drinkers who average more than 1.5 drinks a day lose almost 70 percent more bone than non-drinkers), cigarette smoking, the use of certain drugs, especially steroids (which are commonly used to treat asthma and arthritis), as well as anticoagulants, thyroid medications, aluminum-containing antacids such as Maalox and Mylanta, certain cancer drugs (e.g., methotrexate), and other medications such as the cholesterol-reducer cholestyramine. A diet that is high in fat, caffeine, or salt, but low in calcium (milk and dairy products) places a person at risk for osteoporosis.

Some of the early signs of osteoporosis include back pain and loss of height. You are taller when you arise in the morning and lose height (up to three-quarters of an inch) as your intervertebral discs compress during the day's upright activities. In osteoporosis, because the bone has become weak, small breaks in the spine can occur with an incident as minor as coughing or lifting a bag of groceries. As a result of the gradual accumulated compression of many of these small breaks, people become permanently shorter. If you think you may have lost height, you can use your arm span as a guide. After attaining full growth, most people's height equals their arm span. In African Americans, the arm span is usually slightly greater than the person's height. Curvature of the upper back (dowager's hump) is also a sign of osteoporosis. As noted previously, fractures of the wrist, spine, or hip, as well as loosening or loss of teeth, are frequently found in those who have osteoporosis.

People who have osteoporosis or who are at risk for this disease should be particularly careful about safety factors, both inside and outside the home. Women should not wear high spiked heels. Nor should one bend or lift from the back. Tranquilizers and other sedating drugs should be avoided when feasible. The living environment must be closely monitored for safety hazards.

Any disease that causes poor absorption of calcium in the gastrointestinal tract can produce osteoporosis. Some specific diseases, including hyperparathyroidism, hyperthyroidism, or immobilization from whatever cause, also lead to osteoporosis. Risk factors for osteoporosis are summarized in Table 2-1.

DIAGNOSIS

The onset of osteoporosis can be extremely slow, and the person who has osteoporosis can be symptom-free for some time. Although the disease may be discovered incidentally on an x-ray taken for another reason (at least 30 percent of total bone mass must have been lost), usually the first indication that someone is suffering from osteoporosis is a fracture that results from minimal exertion.

The common sites of fracture have been mentioned, but more should be said concerning vertebral fractures, because they are most common in this condition. Patients with a backbone break usually experience severe pain, which may persist for longer than three months. Wedging collapse of the involved vertebrae (Figure 2-1) can result in loss of height and the so-called dowager's hump mentioned previously. Hip fractures increase with age as bone becomes thinner, with approximately a 1 percent rate of increase per year in those who are older than 75. Osteoporosis is the leading cause of hip fractures that result in significant disability and even death in the elderly; 30 percent of women aged 75 will incur a fracture of

TABLE 2-1.   Risk Factors for Osteoporosis
❑ Increasing age
❑ Female gender
❑ White or Asian race
❑ Early menopause
❑ Small-boned with thin build
❑ Family history of osteoporosis
❑ Fair skin and blue eyes
❑ Few or no children
❑ Chronically low calcium intake
❑ Lack of exercise
❑ Cigarette smoking
❑ Alcohol consumption
❑ High caffeine intake
❑ Corticosteroid treatment
❑ High protein intake
❑ Use of aluminum-containing antacids
❑ High salt intake
❑ Excess thyroid hormone
❑ Restricted mobility
❑ Acromegaly
❑ Hypogonadism
❑ Anorexia nervosa
❑ Jaundice
❑ Malabsorption syndromes
❑ Severe malnutrition
❑ Carcinoma
❑ Certain connective tissue disorders
❑ Certain bone marrow disorders
❑ The use of certain drugs, such as heparin, phenytoin, phenobarbital, methotrexate, cholestyramine
❑ Chronic obstructive pulmonary disease
❑ Chronic nerve disease; diabetes; chronic renal disease; rheumatoid arthritis
❑ History of nontraumatic fracture

either the hip, the thigh bone next to the knee, or a vertebra, osteoporosis being a major contributing factor to such injury. Many hip fracture patients never resume normal activities, and almost 20 percent die within one year after their fracture.

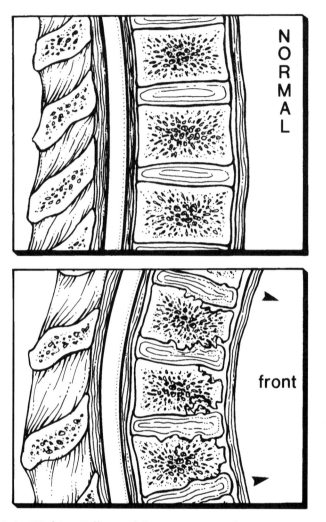

FIGURE 2-1   Wedging Collapse of Osteoporotic Vertebrae

This mortality figure is higher than in patients who suffer a heart attack.

Approximately 80 percent of the mass of the skeleton is cortical bone. However, the spine is only 30 percent cortical bone; the rest is trabecular. As discussed in Chapter 1, the ratio of surface area to volume in trabecular bone is much higher than in compact bone. Trabecular bone has approximately eight times the remodeling rate of its compact counterpart. These features make the trabecular bone of the spine a sensitive indicator of lost bone mass, and several specialized techniques have been developed to measure this.

❏ Quantitative computed tomography is a noninvasive test that does not require ingesting or injecting any material, utilizes a standard CT scanner available at almost any hospital, and is very accurate in detecting osteoporosis of the vertebrae.
❏ Dual photon absorptiometry measures bone density with gamma ray beams. It also is noninvasive, does not require the introduction of any foreign substance into the body, and is generally accepted as a reliable gauge of bone mass.
❏ Dual energy x-ray absorptiometry, single photon absorptiometry, and radiographic absorptiometry are yet other imaging techniques to quantitate bone mass.
❏ Bone densitometry analysis is useful for predicting future fracture risk.
❏ Osteomark is a urine test that measures human bone resorption, allowing physicians to diagnose accelerated bone loss.
❏ A bone biopsy after labeling with tetracycline, an antibiotic taken by mouth, is another way to diagnose osteoporosis and distinguish it from other diseases (e.g., osteomalacia) that weaken bone.

PREVENTION

The best treatment of any disease is prevention, and the best insurance against the complications of osteoporosis is to build strong bone and keep it that way. Plenty of exercise and adequate calcium intake during the years of growth and early adulthood will ensure that bones will be at their peak mass when resorption takes over. Thus, the key is to achieve peak bone density during the time in your life when your body is building your skeleton. You only have until approximately age 25 to do that. By age 35, bone formation continues, but bone loss begins. Calcium and vitamin D supplementation have been noted to stop steroid-induced bone loss. Other drugs such as

Fosamax may also be used in patients who require long-term, low-dose oral steroid therapy.

Postmenopausal bone loss can be decelerated by replacing lost hormones. At the same time, it is crucial to continue to stay physically active, ensure adequate calcium intake, avoid risk factors, and learn to live safely to prevent fractures.

As mentioned previously, estrogen deficiency is an important cause of osteoporosis. As long ago as 1940 researchers realized that ovarian function was a contributing factor in this disease. Estrogen replacement therapy in women can often be successful in inhibiting osteoporosis, because the bone-resorbing cells contain estrogen receptors and estrogen reduces the rate of bone resorption.

Treatment with estrogen seems to be definitely indicated in women who have had a surgically induced menopause. However, misgivings remain about giving estrogen to otherwise healthy postmenopausal women because of the possible association of estrogens with breast and uterine cancer. Some study results have shown that administering estrogen increases the risk of breast cancer, but this is a modest risk— approximately a 30 percent or less increase after 15 years of therapy. Other studies have found no increase in the risk of breast cancer. As high as an eightfold increase in the risk of uterine cancer with estrogen therapy has been documented by several investigations. However, the incidence of uterine cancer is normally very small, approximately one per 1,000 women, so that an eightfold increase is a rate of only eight per 1,000. This cancer appears to be low grade and highly curable. The evidence to date suggests that this danger can be reduced by administering the hormone progestin in conjunction with estrogen. This combined therapy also may protect against breast cancer.

Finally, there is evidence that replacement therapy also protects patients against heart attacks. In fact, some experts even recommend that *every* women should receive estrogen replacement therapy after menopause to protect against not only osteoporosis but also coronary artery disease, unless there is good medical reason not to do so, such as a history of breast or uterine cancer, phlebitis, or active liver disease. Women who have high blood pressure, diabetes, or significant fluid retention may also be advised against taking estrogen. For the average woman, one estrogen pill by itself is prescribed for the first 16 days of the month, and estrogen and progesterone together from day 17 to day 25. No medication is taken on the remaining days, and during this time there may be some withdrawal bleeding. This schedule may vary according to the individual. There are also combinations of drugs, such as Prempro (premarin [estrogen] plus progesterone), which is taken daily without a break.

In order to be effective, estrogen replacement involves long-term therapy. It is often recommended for at least 10 to 12 years and may continue for a lifetime. Recent studies indicate that women who began taking estrogen 18 years after menopause and had been on the hormone for an average of more than nine years had virtually the same bone density as those who began therapy around the time of menopause and had been taking the hormone for an average of 20 years. The important thing seems to be not duration of treatment but remaining on estrogen replacement therapy once it has been started.

If a woman is at high risk when she reaches menopause, she might want to consider starting estrogen therapy immediately. If she is not at especially high risk for osteoporosis or heart disease, she may believe that she has no compelling reason to begin estrogen therapy and can wait before making the decision. If she has a family history of breast cancer, it may be prudent to wait 10 years or more before starting estrogen replacement therapy.

The benefits of hormone replacement include not only the prevention of bone loss, but also the reduction of menopausal symptoms such as hot flashes, moodiness, loss of sleep, excessive perspiration, and drying of the mucosa of the vagina. Estrogens also lower cholesterol levels. However, no treatment is without its downside. Some of the side effects of hormone replacement include breast tenderness and fluid retention. There is a slightly increased risk of gallbladder disease and high blood pressure. Some women resume monthly menstruation, although they are not fertile.

It would be rash of me as a doctor to recommend any treatment for a reader whom I had not seen and assessed personally. Therefore, if you are interested in estrogen therapy, you should consult your own physician to see if hormone replacement is appropriate for you.

TABLE 2-2. How Much Calcium Do You Need?	
Population Group	*Milligrams Per Day*
Children*	
Birth to 6 months	360
6 months to 1 yr	540
1–10 yr	800
10–18 yr	1,200
Pregnant or nursing women*	
<18 yr	2,000
≥19 yr	1,400
Other adults#	
Premenopausal women	1,000
Estrogen-treated women	1,000
Postmenopausal women	1,500
Men <50 years	1,000
>50 years	1,500

* Recommended dietary allowances developed by the National Academy of Sciences, National Research Council.
\# 1983 National Institutes of Health Consensus Development Conference statement on osteoporosis.

There is no evidence that calcium intake above the recommended daily dietary allowance (Table 2-2) is beneficial in preventing or treating osteoporosis. No protection against osteoporosis is gained from higher dietary calcium and such intake may place the patient at increased risk for kidney stones. However, many people do not include adequate calcium in their diet (the average consumption of soft drinks is twice that of milk, and many soft drinks contain a high level of phosphorus, which can impair calcium absorption), and for these individuals oral suplementation is necessary.

Tables 2-2 and 2-3 list the recommended daily dietary calcium intake and some common food sources of this mineral. If you cannot tolerate dairy products because of a lactose intolerance, there are many other foods from which you can get calcium.

If you require a calcium supplement, always check the number of milligrams of elemental calcium contained per pill. This is usually 250 to 500 mg. The highest level of elemental calcium (40 percent) is found in calcium carbonate, which is

TABLE 2-3   **Sources of Calcium**

DAIRY FOODS	Milligrams of calcium
Milk, 1 cup	280–347
Buttermilk	285
Chocolate	280
Malted	347
Whole	291
1% lowfat	300
2% lowfat	297
Skim, med	302
Cheeses	77–337
American, pasteurized process, 1 oz	174
Blue, 1 oz	150
Brick, 1 oz	191
Caraway, 1 oz	191
Cheddar, 1 oz	204

CHEESE FOODS	
American, pasteurized process, 1 oz	163
Swiss, pasteurized process, 1 oz	205
Colby, 1 oz	194
Cottage, 2% lowfat, 1/2 cup	77
Edam, 1 oz	207
Monterey, 1 oz	212
Mozzarella, part skim, 1 oz	207
Muenster, 1 oz	203
Ricotta, part skim, 1/2 cup	337
Swiss, 1 oz	272
Milkshakes	396–457
Chocolate, 10.6 fl oz	396
Vanilla, 11 fl oz	457
Frozen desserts, 1/2 cup	88–137
Ice cream	88
Ice milk, hardened	88
Ice milk, soft serve	137
Yogurts, lowfat, 1 cup	345–415
Flavored	389
Fruit	345
Plain	415
Pudding, chocolate, 1/2 cup	133

SEAFOOD AND LEGUMES	
Beans, dried, cooked, 1 cup	90
Oysters, raw, 7–9	113
Salmon, with bones, 3 oz	167
Sardines, with bones, 3 oz	372

TABLE 2-3   *(Continued)*

SEAFOOD AND LEGUMES	Milligrams of calcium
Shrimp, canned, 3 oz	99
Tofu, processed with calcium sulfate, 4 oz	145
FRUITS AND VEGETABLES	
Bok choy, fresh, cooked, 1/2 cup	79
Collards, fresh, cooked, 1/2 cup	74
Kale, frozen, cooked, 1/2 cup	90
Mustard greens, frozen, cooked, 1/2 cup	75
Spinach, fresh, cooked, 1/2 cup	122
Turnip greens, fresh, cooked, 1/2 cup	99
WHOLE GRAINS	
Cornbread, 2-1/2 × 2-1/2 × 1-5/8 inches	90
Pancakes, 4″ diameter, 2	116
Waffle, 4-1/2 × 4-1/2 × 5/8 inches	120
MISCELLANEOUS	
Cheese pizza, 1/4 of 14″ pie	288
Chili con carne with beans, canned, 1 cup	82
Custard, baked, 1/2 cup	148
Macaroni and cheese, 1/2 cup	181
Soups made with milk, 1 cup	
Cream of mushroom	179
Cream of tomato	159
Spaghetti, meatballs, tomato sauce,	
and cheese, 1 cup	124
Taco, beef	174
Molasses, blackstrap, 1 tbsp	137

CALCIUM SUPPLEMENTS	% of supplement that is calcium
Calcium carbonate	40
Calcium chloride	36
Calcium lactate	13
Calcium gluconate	9
Bone meal	31
Dolomite	22
Oyster shell	28

derived from oyster shells. Some organic supplies of calcium have undesirably high levels of lead. A safe source is the familiar Tums antacid tablet, which is pure calcium carbonate (and also salt-free).

As shown in Figure 2-2, vitamin D is necessary for the absorption of calcium. The high occurrence of *osteomalacia* (*osteon* = bone + *malacia* = softness) in Bedouin Arab women, who are clothed so that only their eyes are exposed to sunlight, is a striking example of this fact. Ancient documents compared the hard skull of Egyptians, who shaved their hair and wore little clothing, with the softer skulls of Persians, who dressed in turbans and heavy wraps.

The recommended daily allowance of vitamin D is 400–600 I.U. This can be obtained from drinking a quart of vitamin D–

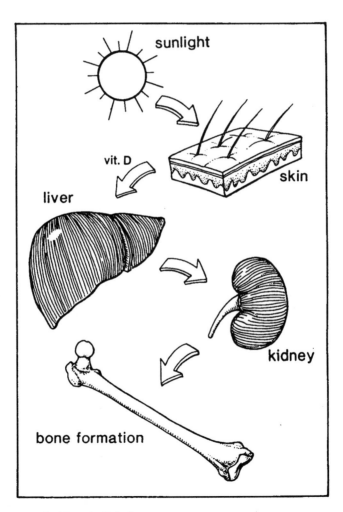

FIGURE 2-2   The Vitamin D Pathway

supplemented milk, taking an average multivitamin pill or a single vitamin D pill, or exposing an area of skin the size of the face to sunshine for an hour. Do not take too much vitamin D; too much of this nutrient can be harmful, causing rarefaction of bone and increased calcium in the blood with deposition in the soft tissues of the body.

Physical activity is a significant factor in increasing bone mass in the young, and exercise is important in maintaining bone integrity in middle and old age. Tennis players, for example, have 20 percent greater bone mass than nonathletes of the same weight. Any exercise is beneficial but weight-bearing activities are best. Of course, those exercises that put the spine and extremities at risk for fracture or other injury must be avoided.

You should check with your personal physician before starting a new exercise program. Body-building exercise should be supervised. Any time you experience pain, you must stop. Walking is an excellent activity that is available to almost everyone at any age. Improving the strength of the quadriceps, the muscles in the front of the upper thigh, is of particular value, because strong quadriceps help prevent falls that can result in broken bones. You will keep the quadriceps in shape by strength-training exercises, such as knee extensions while seated, as well as isometric exercises. Aerobic exercises are especially good for younger people but should be approached cautiously by the elderly.

"Stairmaster" exercising is excellent for cardiac conditioning. The technique and apparatus were developed after a study showed that workers in service vocations who walked up several flights of stairs each working day were at significantly less risk for heart attack. All other factors being equal, it has been estimated that every stair you walk up adds four seconds to your life. A classic study comparing London bus drivers, who sat all day, to conductors, who walked up and down the stairs of the British double-decker buses, found that the conductors lived longer than the drivers. Heavy "stairwalking," however, particularly on a machine that is keyed for resistance, may overload severely osteoporotic hip bones.

Variety is important in any program of physical training as it ensures active use of the entire body and helps keep the participant interested in a daily exercise schedule.

EXERCISE FOR PATIENTS WITH OSTEOPOROSIS

SAFE EXERCISES

- ❏ Gentle floor exercises
- ❏ Riding a stationary cycle
- ❏ Swimming and other exercise in water
- ❏ Dancing. Walking

UNSAFE EXERCISES

- ❏ Heavy aerobic exercise
- ❏ Weight lifting
- ❏ Any exercise that causes back flexion
- ❏ Jumping
- ❏ Jogging
- ❏ Contact sports
- ❏ Bicycle riding
- ❏ Ice skating
- ❏ Skiing
- ❏ Horseback riding

QUADRICEPS STRENGTHENING KNEE MUSCLE EXERCISES

1. Lie on your back on a firm, flat surface, keeping your knee perfectly straight and stiff (180°). Lift the leg as high as possible. Slowly return the leg to the resting position. Relax momentarily.

You should feel tension in the muscles of the front of the thigh during this exercise. Do as many straight leg lifts as possible the first day. Gradually increase the number you can perform by adding one repetition each succeeding day to a maximum of 50 lifts. Continue with 50 lifts daily. Proceed slowly; you may feel fatigue but should not experience pain.

2. Comfortably seated with a shoe on, hook the foot of the involved knee under a desk, sofa, chair, or other piece of furniture that is too heavy to lift. Keeping the knee perfectly straight and stiff, attempt to lift the furniture, exerting a maximal effort, and slowly counting to six. Relax. During the exercise, tension should be felt in the muscles of the front of the thigh. Next, bend the knee approximately 30°, and repeat the exercise. Finally, bend the knee approximately 60°, and repeat the exercise.

These are isometric exercises. The knee should not move during the six-second maximal contracture. Each exercise is to be performed only once during an exercise period. Repeat these isometric exercises three times each day.

The diet should include adequate but not excessive protein and salt. The protein and phosphorus contained in red meat increase calcium loss in the urine. Every extra gram of protein beyond what the body requires for normal growth and maintenance prevents the storage of 1 mg of calcium. Fish and fowl are better sources of protein; they also contain less fat and cholesterol than red meat. Excess fiber reduces absorption of calcium from the intestine. Caffeine also increases loss of calcium, so people lose a considerable amount of calcium if they drink coffee or cola in excess.

TREATMENT

Several experimental treatments for osteoporosis are currently being investigated, including calcitonin, sodium fluoride, and ADFR, or "coherence" therapy.

The hormone calcitonin is a potent inhibitor of bone resorption and is currently being used to treat osteoporosis. Miacilin nasal spray, a synthetic version of salmon calcitonin, has been used as a second-line therapy in women with low bone mass who are at least five years past menopause.

Attention was first drawn to sodium fluoride when osteoporosis was discovered to be lower in areas where fluoride intake was high. Sodium fluoride is effective because it incorporates fluoride into the mineral crystals of bones, rendering the crystalline structure more stable. Newly formed bone that uses the more stable crystals appears to be stronger, and there seems to be a lower incidence of fracture in patients treated with sodium fluoride. Fluoride, however, has some undesirable side effects, including gastrointestinal upset, occasional ulcers, and sometimes joint stiffness. Furthermore, excessively high doses may be toxic. The newer forms of slow-release fluoride seem to build stronger bone without significant gastrointestinal symptoms.

Parathyroid hormone given intermittently has been used to stimulate bone formation. Some recent advances in osteoporosis research include the finding that bone mass increases in teenage girls can be enhanced by supplementation with 500 mg calcium citrate maleate per day. If the increase in total bone mass persists to skeletal maturity, approximately 50 percent of future osteoporotic fractures might be prevented. A daily dose of 5 mg of Risedronate (a nonhormonal agent) prevents bone loss and increases bone mass in early postmenopausal women. Reloxifen, an estrogen substitute, is in the pipeline for approval by the Food and Drug Administration.

Postmenopausal women with osteoporosis experienced 29 percent fewer fractures of the hip compared with patients given a placebo when they were treated with a nonhormonal medication known as alendronate (brand name Fosamax, one of a group of compounds originally used to prevent calcium-based scale in steam boilers). Fosamax is taken orally but only approximately 1 percent is absorbed. These and other drugs are under investigation. There are some areas of contention regarding their ultimate value in the management of osteoporosis that should be resolved over time.

Activate-**D**epress-**F**ree-**R**epeat (ADFR or coherence therapy) relies on the theory that the action of the bone-resorbing cells (osteoclasts) is invariably followed by a local reaction from bone-forming cells (osteoblasts). Bone is locally remodeled by these cell groups. The treatment involves activation of the separate cell populations coherently, depressing the resorption and freeing the osteoblasts to form bone. The therapy is then repeated. How is this done? Phosphates are sometimes used to activate cell populations, and calcitonin and a drug called sodium diphosphonate have been used in an attempt to depress the osteoclasts. The effectiveness of ADFR has been touted but the treatment is still controversial.

Fractures of the wrist heal in approximately three weeks, although it may require six months to restore near total function of this joint. Spinal fractures heal in approximately six to twelve weeks but it may take several years for complete functional recovery. A hip fracture is the most serious, because it involves hospitalization, surgery, and rehabilitation with at best anywhere up to six months' loss of independence, and at worst a fatal end result.

Although one might have osteoporosis, its effects can be minimized. The use of a conservative program of back care (see Chapter 9) will aid in maintaining good spinal posture and if not avoiding at least minimizing vertebral fracture.

Common sense precautions concerning safety can prevent injury to osteoporotic bone. Sedative drugs should be avoided.

CASE REPORT: OSTEOPOROSIS

Mary G. was 68 years old. She was widowed, subsisted on social security benefits, and lived alone. Mary was petite and had very thin bones. She did not smoke or drink but drank several cups of coffee each day. Because she cooked only for herself, her meals were often far from adequate. Mary had a daughter who lived out of state. Mary's mother and two aunts had a history of osteoporosis.

One hot summer day Mary bent over to open a jammed window. She felt a sudden pain in her mid-back that took her breath away. She managed to call her doctor, who arranged for her to be taken to the hospital emergency ward by ambulance. An x-ray revealed a compression fracture of the lower spine. She was admitted to the hospital, where severe osteoporosis was confirmed by dual photon absorptiometry.

Mary was given pain medication and mobilized as quickly as possible. Her vertebral fracture was managed with an appropriate back support. She received counseling from the hospital nutritionist, who instructed her in a well-balanced diet containing adequate natural calcium, modest protein, and low fiber. She was placed on a calcium supplement and vitamin D. Mary was counseled to get sunshine on her face for at least one hour a day when possible. She was also instructed in a weight-bearing exercise program appropriate for her age and ability.

Her status will be closely observed, and if necessary she may be placed on medication such as estrogens or fluoride at a future time. Meanwhile, she has been cautioned to rearrange her apartment with an emphasis on personal safety so as not to inadvertently trip or fall.

Mary G. realizes that she can live comfortably and safely with her osteoporosis by following her physician's advice and preventing further injury.

Shoes that give good support should be worn. Hand rails are a necessity, and all walking areas must be well lit. Proper lifting and bending habits should be cultivated. It is wise not to bend from the back, only from the knees. Objects that weigh more than five to ten pounds should not be lifted. A person at risk for osteoporosis must not use stools, ladders, or chairs to reach high places. Frequently used items should be kept in closets and kitchen cupboards within easy reach, rather than on inaccessible shelves. Walkways should be kept free of clutter and obstacles. All loose wires and electrical cords must be tucked away, and floors and stairways should be kept in good repair. A safety check of the living environment will go a long way toward precheck of the living environment will go a long way toward preventing accidents that can cause fractures in osteoporotic bone.

So, you see, osteoporosis is a condition that can often be prevented and usually curtailed through proper diet, exercise, and living habits. Hormone replacement is available when indicated, and various other medical treatments, although somewhat experimental, can be used when necessary. The National Osteoporosis Foundation offers osteoporosis prevention and treatment information. To order a general information packet, you can write to the National Osteoporosis Foundation, Department MQ, P.O. Box 96616, Washington, D.C. 20077.

QUESTIONS AND ANSWERS ABOUT OSTEOPOROSIS

Q: What foods have a negative effect on calcium metabolism in the body?

A: Fiber decreases intestinal absorption of calcium, whereas protein increases its urinary loss. Caffeine increases both intestinal and urinary loss of calcium. Sodium also increases urinary loss of calcium, whereas phosphorus increases intestinal loss but decreases urinary loss.

Q: What are some of the effects of inadequate calcium intake other than osteoporosis?

A: Inadequate dietary calcium may be an important cause of high blood pressure. Some cases of colon cancer may be brought on by low calcium in the diet. High-calcium diets leave unabsorbed calcium in the food residue that reaches the colon, and this calcium can neutralize irritant substances that may bring out a latent potential for colon cancer. A receding jaw makes denture fitting difficult. A low-calcium diet can aggravate this problem, and calcium supplementation can minimize it.

Q: Is it possible to take in too much calcium?

A: It *is* possible to abuse calcium (which can form kidney stones), but many people consume as much as 10 times the amount of calcium that a typical middle-aged American gets without difficulty. A calcium intake of up to 2,500 mg is safe for almost everyone. It is better to get more calcium than we need than to risk calcium deficiency with all its problems.

Q: Is there any danger in drinking too much milk?

A: People are concerned about the lactose, calories, and cholesterol in dairy products. In fact, dairy products are low in cholesterol, and only fresh or powdered milk is problematic for those who are lactose intolerant. Also, lowfat milk has fewer calories than you might imagine.

Q: How do some youngsters set themselves up for osteoporosis later in life?

A: Eighty-five percent of young women do not get enough calcium. "Thin is in," and most young girls associate calcium intake with milk fat and becoming fat, so they do not drink milk. The long-term effects of shortchanging one's bone bank during development are not easily reversed.

Q: Can high-frequency sound waves be used to evaluate osteoporosis?

A: A new bone scanning device called the *Sahara* uses ultrasound to measure the density of bone in the heel. The test is simple and less expensive than other ways for scanning bone. This method is not very precise in predicting fractures of the spine and hips because it does not measure bone density in those areas. However, it should prove to be useful as a screening tool.

Q: What is raloxifene?

A: Raloxifene (brand name Evista) is a selective estrogen receptor modulator that is used for the prevention of osteoporosis. In addition to safeguarding bone, raloxifene, like estrogen, might also protect the heart by lowering levels of "bad" LDL (low-density lipoprotein) cholesterol, as well as fibrinogen, which is another heart disease risk factor. This is important because heart disease kills almost seven times as many women as breast cancer in the 55 and over age group. Although estrogen stimulates breast and uterine cell growth, which increases the risk of cancer, raloxifene does not appear to do this. This "designer estrogen" is not for women who have not yet reached menopause or for those who have early menopausal symptoms. Postmenopausal women should think seriously about raloxifene as prevention against osteoporosis. However, it is not entirely risk-free. In rare cases, it has caused blood clots in the legs.

Q: Are there any natural remedies for osteoporosis?

A: Some alternative treatments may offer relief. These include vitamin B_6, vitamin E, primrose oil, ginseng, folate, and phytoestrogens, which are natural estrogens found in soy (including tofu), peas, beans, and flaxseed. Because the amount of active hormone in these sources varies, you should talk to your doctor before using them.

3

Arthritis

You can't turn back the clock, but you can wind it up again.

Bonnie Prudden

By now you should realize that bone is a system that is "user friendly." It adapts, repairs, and remodels easily. However, it ages like the rest of the body, and arthritis cannot usually be avoided, at least not the "normal" aging degeneration of joints. Nonetheless, as with osteoporosis, something can be done about this condition. This chapter surveys the subject of arthritis and tells you how to manage it.

THE JOINTS OF THE BODY

Our joints permit movement, but in doing so they often subject themselves to considerable stress and strain. Joints are stabilized by fibrous structures called *ligaments* and are continuously lubricated to offset friction. Joints are lined with *cartilage* (Latin = gristle). Cartilage is composed mainly of a protein called collagen, which is embedded in a firm gel and is thus more flexible than bone. Cartilage lacks blood vessels and is nourished by diffusion from the fluid found in the joint.

All joints are leverage systems. The bones are the lever arms, the joint is the fulcrum, and muscles apply forces that lift the weight of the body or extremity. Because the effectiveness of a lever is a function of both the length of the lever arm and the force applied, people of identical build can have different strengths if their muscles are inserted closer or farther from the fulcrum of their joints.

The ends of bones at synovial joints are separated by a narrow space (the joint cavity) that permits movement. The joint is surrounded by a capsule composed of fibrous tissue. This structure is flexible enough to permit movement but strong enough to prevent dislocation. A thin synovial membrane lines this capsule and secretes synovial fluid, which lubricates the joint (synovia—from *syn* (Greek) = together + *ovum* (Latin) = an egg; thus, the fluid is sticky, like egg white). Joints are lubricated either by "weeping lubrication," in which the synovial fluid absorbed by the cartilage is pressed out when the joint surfaces touch, or by "boosted lubrication," in which the articular cartilage absorbs some molecules of the synovial fluid, allowing molecular mucous compounds to remain behind and lubricate the joint.

Large joints such as the knee and hip are surrounded by *bursal sacs* (Greek: *bursa,* meaning a purse). These bursae act as pads to ease friction between tendons and ligaments on bones. Synovial fluid can be found in these sacs. Inflammation due to pressure, either acute or chronic, can lead to pain and swelling in a bursa. The bursitis that ensues can be treated by anti-inflammatory medications, either injected or taken orally, aspiration of the fluid, and by surgical removal of the offending bursa in severe cases.

Joints have a variety of designs that allow appropriate motion at any body segment. Two major ball and socket joints are the hip and the shoulder. The hip is the deepest joint of the body, with the ball-shaped head of the thigh bone closely fitted into the socket or *acetabulum* (Latin = vinegar cup) of the pelvis. This makes for a very strong and stable joint. The shoulder also has a ball and socket configuration, but it is shallow, thus sacrificing strength for an increased range of motion. These design principles accommodate the need of the body for stability for the standing and walking functions of the hip as well as the range of motion necessary for the many tasks the arms must perform.

The knee is the largest joint in the body. It is basically a hinge joint, but it also rolls and glides as we move. Because the knee bears large loads and is subject to severe stresses, it is stabilized by ligaments on either side as well as by a pair of crossed ligaments inside the joint itself. In addition, several crescent-shaped cartilaginous wedges act as shock absorbers. These *menisci* (Latin = half-moon) permit easy gliding at the knee and also cushion the pounding to which this joint is subjected. Repair of torn menisci accounts for a high percentage of all knee surgery. Such injuries are most common in contact sports, such as football, in which direct blows and twisting of the knee with the foot fixed result in crushing of the menisci and tears of the ligaments of the knee. Because the knee is so frequently injured, I have devoted an entire chapter (Chapter 11) to this important joint. In that chapter we talk in some detail about its anatomy and its injuries.

ARTHRITIS: SOME GENERAL REMARKS

The word *arthritis* means inflammation of a joint (*arthr* = joint; *itis* = inflammation). The signs of arthritis have been identified in the bones of dinosaurs as well as in those of contemporary mammals. Animals that have a cartilaginous skeleton, such as sharks, are protected from arthritis.

There are more than 100 different forms of arthritis. As many as 40 million people in the United States have one type or another, with a projected prevalence of 60 million by the year 2020. Osteoarthritis of the knee alone accounts for as much disability in older Americans as conditions such as diabetes, heart disease, hip fracture, and depression. It is a serious reason for lost time at work and causes significant disability, resulting in the hospitalization of more than 500,000 people each year. Arthritis is mainly a disease of adults, but there are childhood forms; arthritis affects 250,000 young people under 16 years of age in the United States.

In many instances the word *arthritis* is a misnomer. Inflammation is part of the body's normal reaction to any insult. It represents one of the body's natural defenses at work, attempting to repair a problem of injury or disease. This often results in swelling, stiffness, redness, tenderness, and pain. These signs are present in some forms of arthritis but may be absent in others, in which the condition is mainly one of degeneration. At the same time, arthritis can be primarily infectious due to a variety of bacterial (or even viral) agents, including gonorrhea and tuberculosis. The first signs of infectious arthritis may be fever and chills followed by a swollen, painful joint.

Some conditions of the soft tissues (ligaments, fascia, tendons, bursae) are "cousins" of arthritis that frequently mimic it. These disorders fall under the general rubric of soft tissue rheumatism (from the Greek word *rheumatismos,* meaning suffering from a flux). They can affect young people as well as older individuals, and it has been estimated that there are 12 million sufferers in the United States alone. Cartilage in locations other than a joint (for instance, between the ribs and the sternum) can also become inflamed, mimicking arthritis. Muscles also can be irritated and painful. This is called *myositis* or *myalgia* (*myo* = muscular, *algia* = pain) as a part of an arthritic condition or in isolation, leading to symptoms that may be confused with arthritis. Because pain is the "alarm system" of the body, it is important to make as exact a diagnosis as possible and not just "take something for the pain." Anyone who plays doctor and self-medicates himself for undiagnosed pain beyond a reasonable time has a fool for a patient and a damn fool for a doctor.

Some of the conditions in this group of soft tissue diseases are tendinitis, bursitis, capsulitis, ligamentitis, fasciitis, and fibrositis. These are all considered in detail in other chapters but are mentioned here because they are frequently included in the differential diagnosis of arthritis. Inflammation of the soft tissues can occur because of an infection or excessive use of the part involved. The names given to these painful conditions reflect the many occupations, sports, and recreations that are affected. Consider ballet toe, dancer's hip, golfer's elbow, housemaid's or jumper's knee, Pac-man tendinitis, tennis elbow, marcher's heel, bowler's thumb, weaver's bottom, and so forth.

Because of the close connection between the psyche (mind) and the soma (body), arthritic and nonarthritic pain can be exaggerated or even caused by an agitated mental state. When there is no organic cause of pain and disability, the condition is called pure psychogenic rheumatism.

Ankylosing spondylitis is an inflammation where the soft tissues attach to bone. It most commonly affects the spine, stiffening and eventually fusing it. Ankylosing spondylitis tends to run in families because of the inheritance of a particular gene.

Polymyalgia rheumatica is a condition of stiffness in the neck, shoulders, and hips that is usually seen in older women.

Pains around the joints occur and often mimic those of arthritis. A particular blood test, the sedimentation rate, is always elevated in this condition. Treatment is low doses of steroids. Therapy must be continued for a long period of time, as the steroids are gradually reduced. It is dangerous to take a patient off steroid medication abruptly, because the body's ability to produce its own steroids is depressed while taking steroids by mouth, and is only gradually re-established as the oral medication is slowly withdrawn.

Reflex sympathetic dystrophy is a malfunction of the sympathetic (autonomic) nervous system that leads to *Sudeck's atrophy* (Sudeck, a German surgeon, first described the condition in 1900), which can occur with even a minor injury to a joint. This condition is caused by underuse of the involved body part (foot, hand, and so forth) due to pain, which leads to decreased circulation, thinning of the involved bones, and weakness and contracture of soft tissue structures in the area. Treatment is to blockade the sympathetic nervous system with local anesthetic blocks, to control pain through oral medication, and to insist on a vigorous exercise regimen supervised by a physical therapist.

Now, on to the most familiar forms of arthritis, osteoarthritis, rheumatoid arthritis, and gout.

OSTEOARTHRITIS

Osteoarthritis, sometimes called degenerative arthritis, is the most common form of arthritis. It is estimated that 17 million people in the United States have osteoarthritis. It is caused by the breakdown of articular cartilage inside a joint. Cartilage loses its ability to act as a "shock absorber" and little "spurs" can form at the margins of joints. Osteoarthritis occurs as a natural consequence of aging, but it may begin earlier as a result of joint overuse or an injury such as a fracture or repeated sprain. Certain diseases such as diabetes and hypothyroidism predispose one to osteoarthritis. Typically, the major weight-bearing joints are involved, such as the spine, hip, and knee. Osteonecrosis of the knee can mimic osteoarthritis. It is a rather sudden collapse of one of the articular surfaces of the femur at the knee joint that occurs in older people; its cause is not known. Definitive treatment is surgery to either replace the damaged bone with a prosthetic joint or realign the knee to shift weight off the collapsed bone. Occasionally the shoulders, wrists, and elbows can be affected, particularly if these joints have been overused or injured.

Nearly 85 percent to 90 percent of all people over the age of 60 show some signs of osteoarthritis. Although there is no cure, relief may be obtained through the use of drugs, physical therapy, and surgery in selected cases.

The cause of osteoarthritis is not completely known, but some researchers theorize that it may be due to malalignment of the involved joints. The condition also appears to have some hereditary basis and is seen in conditions such as acromegaly, in which an excess of growth hormone causes bony overgrowth and arthritis. The character "Jaws" in the James Bond movies displays such features. The normally smooth cartilage becomes irregular, restricting motion and causing pain on movement. Knobby points of cartilage and bone may develop at the ends of the fingers (Heberden's nodes) or at the middle of the fingers (Bouchard's nodes).

Localized inflammation due to breakdown of cartilage with spillage of irritating chemicals into the joint can cause inflammation in osteoarthritis. Erosion of cartilage then proceeds to expose underlying bone, which results in even more inflammation, pain, and stiffness. Muscles go into spasm and become fatigued. The breakdown of the intervertebral disc may cause pain in the lower back (Figure 3-1), and overgrowth of bone locally can produce pressure on nerves, leading to sciatica. Osteoarthritis of the neck may similarly cause nerve root pressure, with pain spreading to the ear or shoulder. Hip pain can radiate to the buttocks or groin, and knee instability and weakness can cause difficulty, particularly when walking stairs. People with osteoarthritis usually find that stiffness is worse after rest and that their joints loosen up with activity, although some find that stiffness and pain increase as the day goes on. Creaking or grating sounds (crepitus) in the joints may be experienced on movement (Figure 3-2).

Patients suffering from suspected osteoarthritis require a complete medical workup that includes a history and physical examination, x-rays, and occasionally aspiration of joint fluid. Blood tests are necessary to be sure that other types of arthritis are not present, such as gouty arthritis and rheumatoid

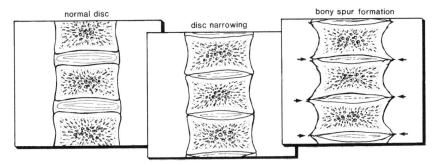

FIGURE 3-1   Disc Degeneration Leading to Arthritis of the Back

arthritis. The blood from patients who have gout contains an overabundance of uric acid, and blood from a patient who has rheumatoid arthritis often reveals a specific rheumatoid factor. Other blood examinations include DNA tests or antinuclear tests. Radiographs in osteoarthritis show joint narrowing due to cartilage loss as well as bony overgrowth (spurs) with thickening of the bones about the involved joints. There may be an excess of synovial fluid in response to joint irritation in osteoarthritis. This fluid typically is not as inflammatory as that found in rheumatoid arthritis.

A variety of drugs are available to treat osteoarthritis pain. Aspirin is a time-proven anti-pain and anti-inflammatory drug. A precursor of aspirin, salicin, found in the bitter leaves of the willow tree, was known to Hippocrates. Aspirin was discovered in 1889 and became available over-the-counter circa 1900. Americans use approximately 175 aspirin tablets per person each year. This amounts to 80 million aspirin a day or 16,000 tons of aspirin each year for the country as a whole. To minimize stomach upset, aspirin is usually taken with food and/or antacids. People who are allergic to aspirin may develop an asthmatic reaction that involves wheezing or shortness of breath. Aspirin decreases the ability of blood to clot (that is why it is taken to prevent heart attacks). Large doses can cause ringing in the ears. Enteric-coated aspirin should not irritate the stomach. It should not be given with milk, however, because milk quickly dissolves the coating. Aspirin should never be taken with either alcohol or vitamin C; such combinations may seriously irritate the gastrointestinal tract.

Nonsteroidal anti-inflammatory drugs (NSAIDs) are a relatively new class of drugs available for the treatment of osteoarthritis. Approximately 300 million prescriptions for NSAIDs are written each year. Although they are often effective, these drugs may have side effects that include stomach upset and kidney or liver damage. The patient taking an NSAID should be closely monitored by his or her physician.

Aspirin is technically an NSAID. Examples of other drugs in this category include piroxicam (Feldene), diclofenate sodium (Voltaren), ibuprofen (Motrin), indomethacin (Indocin), naproxen (Naprosyn), sulindac (Clinoril), tolmetin (Tolectin), diflunisal (Dolobid), oxaprozin (Daypro), and nabumetone (Relafen). Ibuprofen has been available over-the-counter since 1984, naproxen since 1994. The sales of over-the-counter pain relievers last year was $2.67 billion.

Corticosteroids are often useful when they are injected directly into an osteoarthritic joint. The joint is first aspirated (fluid is withdrawn), and the steroid is then injected. Using corticosteroids in this manner can markedly decrease inflammation and pain in joints. However, they should not be used indiscriminately or over a long period of time because of side effects that include fluid retention, increased blood pressure, osteoporosis, gastrointestinal bleeding, weight gain, fat distribution changes, proneness to infections, slow healing of injuries, and cataracts, to mention a few. Muscle relaxants are sometimes useful to decrease muscle spasm. Various liniments that act as counterirritants producing local heat may give temporary relief of pain. Capsaicin cream, a nonprescription drug derived from the pepper plant, can provide analgesia by inhibiting chemical pain transmission.

Every year Americans spend almost $1 billion on unproved arthritis remedies. Many of these are dietary supplements that are not required to undergo the rigorous testing or federal regula-

FIGURE 3-2   The Arthritis Scenario

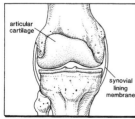
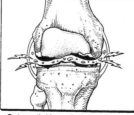
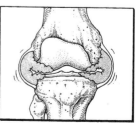

A Healthy Knee Joint

Osteoarthritis–articular cartilage degenerates and fragments

Rheumatoid Arthritis–an inflamed synovial membrane erodes the joint

tion that a drug must go through before the Food and Drug Administration would allow it on the market. The latest fad is a combination of glucosamine and chondroitin sulfate, which, unlike traditional treatments for osteoarthritis that focus on decreasing pain and improving movement of afflicted joints, works to build damaged tissues and halt progression of the disease. For several years veterinarians have used a version of glucosamine (called glucosamine sulfate) to treat osteoarthritis in animals. The effectiveness of these supplements in humans is questioned, however, because most of the studies use reduction of pain as the condition that determines the efficacy of the substance. Because the perception of pain is subjective—typically about 40 percent of patients who try any new treatment experience a reduction of pain due to a powerful placebo effect—measuring it accurately is very difficult.

The person with osteoarthritis must avoid excessive weight gain, which places undue stress on arthritic joints. At the same time, he should maintain general nutrition with a well-balanced, vitamin-supplemented diet. Involved joints may be protected with splints, and walking aids such as canes and crutches can be used. Every five pounds of pressure applied to a cane relieves the supporting leg of 25 pounds of load. The patient should learn to perform his daily activities in the least stressful manner. Devices such as wall brackets in the tub or a raised toilet seat can make day-to-day living more comfortable. Exercise supervised by a physical therapist can increase the range of motion of involved joints, increasing strength and improving function. Resistance and even aerobic exercise can strengthen muscles, so that they are better able to protect joints by absorbing shock and improving stability. Exercise also increases joint flexibility, which lessens pain and decreases the risk of sprains. The joint pressure that occurs with exercise helps cartilage squeeze out waste and soak up nutrients and oxygen. The more a joint is exercised, the healthier it is likely to be.

Cold packs may be used for acute pain, and moist heat often alleviates chronic discomfort. Osteoarthritic hands often respond to warm wax treatments. Ultrasonography and even diathermy have been used with success. Transcutaneous electrical nerve stimulation (TENS) consists of a portable battery wired to pads that attach to the skin. The electrical current stimulates nerves, thereby relieving pain. Acupuncture can also reduce pain in selected cases. A new treatment for osteoarthritis of the knee, the injection of hyaluronic acid to normalize metabolism, is currently being researched.

Finally, surgery may be beneficial for pain that does not respond to conventional therapy. Surgical procedures include tidal irrigation (joint flushing); realignment of the involved joint (now possible with computer assistance to plan and perform the surgery with three-dimensional accuracy); total joint replacement (usually of the hip or knee, although other joints such as fingers, toes, wrists, elbows, shoulders, and ankles may also be replaced); fusion, which permanently holds the bone ends together to prevent motion with attendant pain; or arthroscopic debridement, which involves a "housecleaning" of the affected joint.

CASE REPORT: OSTEOARTHRITIS

Marty S., a 67-year-old retired salesman, experienced increasing stiffness in his hips and knees after rest. As the day wore on, he had to sit frequently to relieve pain in these joints. His fingers were becoming deformed, and the last joints of several fingers were developing tender swellings that were firm to the touch. Marty had been a recreational athlete for most of his life, but pain was preventing him from taking the long walks he so much enjoyed.

After taking his history and giving him a thorough physical examination, Marty's doctor ordered x-rays of his knees, hips, and hands. Findings consistent with osteoarthritis were seen. Blood tests failed to reveal any evidence of infection or rheumatoid arthritis. Marty's uric acid level was normal.

His doctor prescribed an NSAID and advised Marty to take off 15 pounds because he was a bit heavy. Physical therapy treatments were prescribed, including warm whirlpool baths for Marty's hips and knees. He was encouraged to continue an aggressive exercise program but to use a cane for long-distance walking. If this conservative program of management is not successful, he may require injections of cortisone into any joint that is symptomatic. Marty's osteoarthritis will be closely followed. Severe joint destruction in the future could require joint replacement surgery.

RHEUMATOID ARTHRITIS

Rheumatoid arthritis is the second most common form of arthritis, affecting approximately seven million Americans. It has also had some famous sufferers, one of the most notable being the impressionist painter Matisse, whose severe arthritic hand deformities strongly influenced the work of his later years. It initially involves the synovial membrane and is characterized by a chronic (long-lasting) inflammatory disease of joints and other parts of the body (such as the heart or lungs). In rheumatoid arthritis, irritating erosive chemical substances are found in the joint fluid. These are produced by the joint lining, which swells and thickens, eroding and severely damaging the joint surface. The joints most commonly involved are the hands (particularly the first joints of the fingers, which develop a spindle-shaped enlargement), wrists, feet, and ankles, although large weight-bearing joints such as the hips and knees may also be affected. Swelling, pain, deformity, and stiffness are usually present. The disease usually affects many joints at the same time, although there are cases in which only one or two joints are involved. A juvenile form of rheumatoid arthritis can be crippling.

The cause of rheumatoid arthritis is unknown, although it is believed to be an autoimmune disease. This is a condition in which the involved body tissue (particularly the synovial lining of the joints) is the victim of an immune response against itself.

Rheumatoid arthritis is most frequently found in women. It usually affects those who have a fair complexion and red hair. A history of joint swelling, stiffness, and limitation of motion is common. Physical examination reveals swelling and tenderness about the joints, including those of the midportion of the fingers. So-called rheumatoid nodules may appear around joints, particularly the elbow.

Mild anemia is present, the sedimentation rate may be elevated, and blood tests for the disease include those for rheumatoid factors. Radiographs early in the course of the disease reveal only thinning (osteoporosis) of the bone around involved joints, but severe degenerative changes can be seen later. Joint aspiration demonstrates inflammation of the fluid, with cloudiness and the presence of numerous white blood cells. Treatment is similar to that for osteoarthritis, with the addition of other specific medications that include gold and oral corticosteroids. The same precautions given for injectable steroids apply to oral steroids, only more so. Hydroxychloroquine and penicillamine are two other disease-modifying antirheumatic drugs, and immunosuppressive drugs such as azathioprine, cyclophosphamide, cyclosporine, and methotrexate are sometimes given to severe rheumatoid arthritics. Experimental therapies include intravenous gamma globulin (IgG) and interferon, biologic interventions that target specific immune reactions. Side effects from all these medications are many and can be severe. Their use must be closely monitored by a knowledgeable physician. Surgery, including removal of offending synovia but particularly total joint replacement, can return a severely crippled rheumatoid patient to an active life by reducing pain and restoring movement.

Rheumatoid arthritis is best treated by a team of health professionals that includes rheumatologists (arthritis specialists), physical and occupational therapists, social workers, and orthopaedic surgeons.

CASE REPORT: RHEUMATOID ARTHRITIS

Susan L., a 30-year-old woman with a fair complexion and auburn hair, began to notice morning stiffness and pain on motion as well as tenderness in the small joints of her hands. After several weeks, she experienced swelling of her fingers, after which her feet also began to swell and ache. Involvement of her joints was always symmetric. Tender nodules appeared over her elbow joints. During this time, Susan was more fatigued than usual, had lost her appetite, and in fact had lost several pounds in weight. She felt weak and generally achy and stiff.

Susan's doctor took x-rays of her hands, which showed thinning of the bone next to her joints. She was anemic, her sedimentation rate was elevated, and a blood test was positive for rheumatoid factors. A diagnosis of rheumatoid arthritis was made.

Susan was initially managed with high doses of aspirin, taken daily with food. She was placed on a program of physical therapy that included heat, massage, and gentle exercise. Gold therapy was started when her condition did not stabilize. She improved on this regimen and will be observed closely for progress of her disease to other joints.

GOUT

Gout is no joke despite cartoons of a gluttonous aristocrat, his face contorted in pain, his swollen foot elevated on several pillows. It also is small consolation that historically it has afflicted such wise and famous men as Henry VIII, Kubla Khan, Martin Luther, Goethe, Charlemagne, John Milton, Oliver Cromwell,

Isaac Newton, Galileo, Charles Darwin, Theodore Roosevelt, and William Pitt the Elder, to mention but a few. A goutlike disease of uric acid metabolism also affects the Dalmatian breed of pedigree dogs. This ancient disease, once called the rheumatism of the rich and now known to result from a metabolic flaw, is not caused by—only aggravated by—overindulgence in food or drink.

Gouty arthritis is caused by an excess of uric acid in the system. Uric acid is the end product of the breakdown of certain foods. The patient with gout may present with pain in any joint, but most typically the bunion joint of the large toe is painful, red, and swollen. A blood test will show an elevated uric acid, and examination of fluid from an involved joint will reveal uric acid crystals. Occasionally the accumulation of uric acid crystals will cause what is known as a gouty tophus, which sometimes has to be removed surgically.

The word *gout* originates from the Latin: *gutta,* meaning a drop, because the inflammation was supposedly due to the discharge, drop-by-drop, of harmful humors into the joints. It is now known that gout is caused by either too much production or too little excretion of the metabolite uric acid. With its accumulation in or around the affected part (usually a joint), attacks can be triggered by stress—gastronomic, emotional, or physical.

Gout plays no national favorites even though the French claim they have gouté for the taste, whereas the English have gout for the result. However, it does show a strong gender predilection; 95 percent of gout sufferers are men, most of whom are highly achievement-oriented. This striking correlation between gout and prominence (it has been shown statistically that men with high IQs and increased blood uric acid levels are more likely to be leaders) has never been adequately explained. Gout is an ancient disease described in the Bible, "And Esau in the thirty and ninth year of his reign was diseased in his feet, until his disease was exceedingly great: yet in his disease he sought not the Lord, but to the physician. . ." (II Chronicles 16:12). In fact, Aaron's admonition to his sons that they not partake of wine, "else they die," may refer to the association of severe attacks of gout with alcoholic intake.

The patient with gout should be under the supervision of a physician. Advice given usually includes weight reduction and avoiding foods that are high in purines, a metabolic precursor of uric acid; these include organ foods such as liver and kidney as well as foods such as sardines.

Nearly two million Americans suffer from gout. A genetic factor may be involved because some patients with gout have specific enzyme deficiencies that lead to the condition. An acute attack of gout may be precipitated by overindulgence in alcohol, overeating, or psychological or physical tension.

People with gout are well advised to moderate their lifestyle, get plenty of rest and relaxation, and remain under the supervision of a physician who is familiar with the management of the disease. Gout was believed to be due not only to high living (a Spanish proverb says, "Gout is cured by walling up the mouth") but also to lechery. Benjamin Franklin, another notable gout sufferer, wrote, "Be temperate in wine, in eating, girls, and sloth, or the gout will seize you and plague you both" (*Poor Richard's Almanac*, 1734). The father of medicine, Hippocrates, states in his aphorisms, "Eunuchs do not take the gout, nor become bald . . . a young man does not take the gout until he indulges in coition." Although overstated, there seems to be a measure of truth in these observations because the process of gouty inflammation occurs mostly in the presence of male hormones.

Although it can affect any joint, gout usually begins in the great toe. This involvement is called podagra, literally, "a foot attack:"

> Full soon the sad effect of this (port wine)
> his frame began to show
> for that old enemy the gout
> had taken him in toe
> (Thomas Hood, 1799–1845)

The pain is almost unbearable and has been eloquently described by many great authors, including Jonathan Swift:

> Dear, honest Ned is in the gout
> lies rackt with pain, and you without:
> How patiently you hear him groan!
> How glad the case is not your own!

Modern treatment consists of reasonable living habits, including proper diet and moderate exercise, because an episode of gout can be triggered by overweight, as well as by either too little or too much exercise with diminished fluid intake. To abort the acute episode, patients are given certain NSAIDs, cortisone, or colchicine, a drug known to the ancients as both a specific for easing the pain of gout and an assassin's poison that causes violent diarrhea and death. Further attacks can be prevented by drugs that either limit the production of uric acid or encourage its excretion. Some examples are Benemid and Allopurinol.

With all the folklore, it is sometimes difficult to sort fact from fiction, but venery and overeating apart, gout is very real to those who suffer it. And no joking matter!

CASE REPORT: GOUT

Walter M., a 42-year-old, overweight, mail clerk, presented with the sudden onset of pain, swelling, redness, and tenderness at the base of his right great toe. His attack of pain awakened him from a sound sleep in the middle of the night. He had eaten a large dinner, with copious amounts of alcohol before retiring. He described the pain as a violent stretching and tearing alternating with pressure and tightening, and so severe that he could not bear even the weight of the bedsheets on the affected foot.

Radiographs demonstrated arthritis of the great toe, with early cystic changes about the joint, and a blood test revealed a markedly elevated uric acid. The diagnosis of acute gout was made, and Walter was started on colchicine. It took three tablets at hourly intervals before Walter began to sense relief of his pain. After the acute attack had subsided, Walter was managed over the long term on a medication designed to lower his uric acid levels. He was advised to significantly reduce his weight, refrain from eating rich foods (particularly organ meats such as kidney or liver), restrict his alcohol intake and discontinue smoking, get plenty of rest, and try to avoid physical and emotional stress. His gout was easily managed on such a regimen, and he has not had another acute attack.

Finally, a word about offbeat arthritis treatment. Henry VII's physician applied baked ox dung wrapped in cabbage leaves to his swollen joints, and even today the approximately 35 million Americans suffering from arthritis are prime targets for questionable treatments or so-called arthritis cures. The Arthritis Foundation estimates that $950 million is wasted each year on worthless quack remedies. This amounts to $25 spent on unproved treatments for each $1 going toward bona fide research on rheumatic diseases. Such bogus cures take many forms—from copper bracelets to various herbal remedies, with every sort of electrical gadget in between. Not only are these "therapies" useless but, in addition to wasting your money, some of them are downright harmful. All of them delay effective treatment. If in doubt, contact your local Arthritis Foundation office and save yourself a lot of grief. You can reach the National Arthritis Foundation at 1-800-283-7800, or you can visit its World Wide Web site at http://www.arthritis.org, which provides a listing of local chapters as well as general information about arthritis.

The various forms of arthritis, collectively known as the *arthritides*, are common ailments that are seen frequently in any active orthopaedic practice. The only condition seen more often is a broken bone, which we discuss in the next chapter.

QUESTIONS AND ANSWERS ABOUT ARTHRITIS

Q: Does developing arthritis have anything to do with how active or inactive you have been?

A: A lifetime of working heavily or engaging in a rough athletic activity does not mean that you will definitely develop arthritis, and a quiet, inactive life does not necessarily mean that you will not.

Q: Do rheumatoid arthritis and osteoarthritis ever occur together?

A: Rheumatoid arthritis and osteoarthritis frequently occur together because the inflammation secondary to rheumatoid arthritis can produce joint irregularities that subsequently cause osteoarthritis. This is called mixed arthritis.

Q: Is osteoarthritis exclusively a disease of the elderly?

A: No. Although anyone who lives long enough will probably develop osteoarthritis to some extent (some say that one of six Americans has osteoarthritis), many people in their thirties or forties have the disease. In people under 45 years old, osteoarthritis is seen more frequently in men, but more women than men have it after the age of 45.

Q: Can osteoarthritis develop from putting repeated stress on joints?

A: Young people can develop osteoarthritis from activities that are repeatedly hard on their joints. Joe Namath, the great New York quarterback, had an osteoarthritic condition of his knees that resulted from repeated injuries he suffered while playing football. Ballet dancers may develop osteoarthritis in their knees, ankles, or toes. This is caused by the constant unnatural distribution of weight and the stress on impact of landing with full weight on one foot.

Q: How does excessive weight aggravate arthritis?

A: By loading added pressure on joints.

Q: Is heat or cold better for the relief of arthritic pain?

A: Both can be helpful. Heat can relax muscles and improve circulation. Also, a hot tub bath can make your body buoyant, which can provide rest for your joints. For the temporary relief of pain and soreness, cold compresses or an ice pack are good for relieving swelling and decreasing muscle spasm and pain.

Q: Is there a cure for osteoarthritis?

A: Unfortunately, there is no cure for osteoarthritis. However, a treatment plan that includes appropriate exercise and improvement of posture, avoiding those situations that overuse joints, the judicious use of therapeutic measures such as heat and cold, and adherence to a physician's advice including the use of medication and surgery where indicated, can reduce or prevent disability, ease pain and discomfort, and help you to continue your usual activities as independently as feasible for as long as possible.

Q: Are there treatments that, although popular, do not cure arthritis?

A: Yes, indeed. One of these is wearing a copper bracelet. This is based on a false claim that the body absorbs the copper. Another myth is that osteoarthritis can be cured by carrying a horse chestnut on the body or by sitting in an abandoned mine to soak up radiation from uranium. Special diets have been touted, but there is no known diet that can cause, prevent, or cure osteoarthritis. Because the symptoms of osteoarthritis often come and go on their own (spontaneous remission), these cures may sometimes seem to work.

Q: Is dimethylsulfoxide (DMSO) of any value in the treatment of osteoarthritis?

A: DMSO is used commercially as a cleaning solvent and antifreeze chemical. The FDA has not approved the drug for use in treating osteoarthritis. No studies have been done on people with chronic osteoarthritis. Although DMSO has been used in one disease of the urinary tract and is commonly used for veterinary medical purposes, it is potentially dangerous. We must wait for all studies to be completed so that the side effects can be fully known and all danger eliminated before it is used, if indeed it proves beneficial at all.

Q: Are changes in lifestyle sometimes necessary for an arthritic?

A: Yes. One should organize one's life to avoid physical and emotional stress and arrange one's living situation to provide the most efficient and energy-saving ways to perform the tasks of daily living. An occupational therapist can help an arthritic patient to achieve self-sufficiency.

Q: Must sexual relations be curtailed if one has arthritis?

A: There is usually no reason for arthritics not to enjoy a good sex life. Openness on the part of both partners and a willingness to modify sexual technique to accommodate fatigue, pain, and deformity can go a long way toward ensuring a mutually gratifying sex life. It should be remembered that even hugging and touching one's partner can be comforting.

Q: Should arthritics try to live in a hot, dry climate?

A: Although many arthritics find that their arthritis is worse with abrupt weather changes or damp weather, this is not universally so. Moving to a drier climate cannot guarantee improvement in the state of one's arthritis.

Q: How is arthritis linked to psoriasis?

A: The common dermatologic problem of psoriasis can be associated with arthritis, particularly affecting the hands and feet. Unlike rheumatoid arthritis, it usually only affects one side of the body.

Q: What is Reiter's syndrome? Felty's syndrome?

A: Reiter's syndrome is a combination of eye and urinary tract inflammation with arthritis. It follows an infection, often bacterial dysentery and colitis caused by the Shigella or Salmonella organisms. Felty's syndrome is a combination of enlargement of the spleen, low white blood count, and rheumatoid arthritis.

Q: Does repetitive activity promote or accelerate osteoarthritis?

A: In the absence of joint abnormality, physical activity within the limits of comfort and the normal range of motion does not lead to joint injury. Studies comparing runners with sedentary controls have found no difference in the appearance or progression of osteoarthritis between the groups. Incidentally, the development of disability was significantly slower in the runners. Only exercise that subjects joints to abnormal stresses, such as soccer or heavy weightlifting, has been linked to osteoarthritis.

4

Fractures

The broken bone, once set together, is stronger than ever.

John Lyly, Euphues

Although it is light, bone is both flexible and strong. However, it is often injured when pushed beyond its point of resilience. Believe it or not, bone can withstand tension of up to 10 pounds per square inch, but it will often break beyond that point. The technical term for a broken bone is a *fracture* (from the Latin, meaning a break). Despite the common belief (expressed in the quotation heading this chapter) that a fracture heals a bone stronger than it was before being broken, it does not—as strong, yes, but stronger, no.

There are various types and degrees of severity of fractures. Although tensile stress was used in the foregoing example, bone can also fracture as a result of the application of compressive or sheer forces.

The strength of bone and the nature of the forces acting on it change from childhood to old age. These changes occur normally and as a result of disease. Thus, three factors—age, the presence or absence of disease, and the nature of the force—all influence the type and degree of fracture. A fracture may be partial, without complete separation, or it may be complete. In *open fractures*, the broken ends of bone pierce the skin. In a *comminuted fracture*, the bone is splintered into many pieces. Children's bones are springy, like a freshly cut sapling. They often have *greenstick fractures*, due to the elasticity of their bones, which resemble a young twig that can be broken on one side but only bent on the other. Fractures in children heal more rapidly and more surely than those in adults because the growth plate is second only to the skin in its speed of cell regeneration. However, disruption of the epiphyseal (growth) cartilage in a child may cause growth arrest and angular deformity at the joint.

In contrast to children, who often break their bones because of their lively behavior, fractures in the 20 to 50 year age group, especially among men, are often caused by the high energy forces sustained in motor vehicle and work-incurred accidents. The energy generated by these injuries often produces severely displaced fractures associated with massive soft tissue injury.

In older people, fractures can be caused by mild strains acting on osteoporotic bone, as discussed in Chapter 2. These fractures usually occur in cancellous bone rather than in cortical bone. Less common reasons for decreased bone strength are osteomalacia and *osteogenesis imperfecta*, a collagen disease that profoundly affects bone, causing it to become weak and fragile.

Fatigue or stress fractures are seen in athletes, such as fractures of the bones of the foot or lower leg in runners. They can also be seen in older women who have subjected their feet to the rigors of shopping or prolonged standing. They are caused by minimum but repeated trauma to the involved bone. This produces repeated small (micro) fractures, which may eventually develop into a full-fledged bony break.

Various types of fractures have been duplicated experimentally with controlled conditions of loading. These experiments have taught us that bone resists tension less well than compression. We have also learned that a large load may be tolerated if it is slowly applied, but that the same load can break a bone when it is applied rapidly. Fractures of cancellous bone such as a vertebra more often result from compression.

Because bone is a dynamic tissue, physical activity stimulates bone production, particularly when it generates forces in compression. On the other hand, inactivity results in bone resorption.

Except in high energy fracture, vessels and nerves usually escape injury because of their elasticity. Nonetheless, certain fractures are often associated with nerve or vessel damage, such as those about the elbow, knee, and ankle.

Fractures begin to heal at the moment they occur (Figure 4-1). Healing is accomplished through a process of clearing away the broken fragments of bone and depositing new bony tissue. Bleeding from blood vessels in the bone forms a clot (hematoma) shortly after injury. Invasion of this clot by cellular elements forms an organic matrix within which mineral is deposited to create a bridge between the fracture fragments. This bridge is called a *callus* (from the Latin: hard, although it can also mean beam or rafter). Minerals are

FIGURE 4-1   Bone Repair and Remodeling

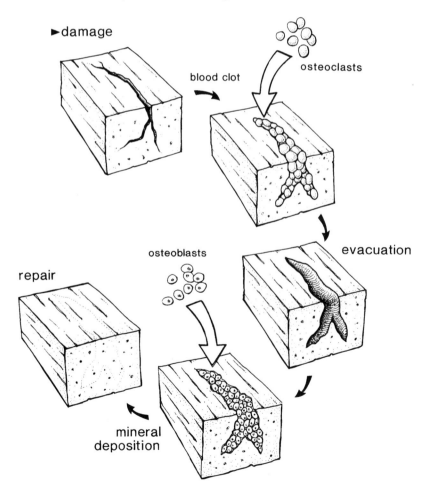

deposited in this bridge, osteoblasts lay down bone, and osteoclasts remodel it.

As one might expect, because of its lesser density, a fracture in cancellous bone usually heals faster than a fracture in its cortical cousin. Thus, a break of the cancellous bone in the upper end of the humerus usually requires one-third or less time to heal than a fracture of the cortical shaft of the same bone. A fracture of the femur (thigh bone) in an infant will heal in four to six weeks, but healing may require as many months in an adult.

Mark Twain called man "a rickety poor sort of thing, always undergoing repairs." Although undoubtedly true, we have developed quite a repertory to help heal broken bones. Common to all systems of fracture treatment is the principle of reducing and immobilizing the fracture. *Reduction* involves restoring the broken bone as closely as possible to the anatomic configuration it had before fracture. *Immobilization* involves preventing motion until the break heals. The treatment of a fracture was reported in Ezekiel (30:21), ". . . son of man, I have broken the arm of Pharaoh, King of Egypt; and lo, it hath not been bound up to be healed, to put a roller, that it be bound up and wax strong, that it hold the sword. . . ." The Egyptians used gauze stiffened with dried egg white for splintage. Native Americans used birch bark splints.

Although a fracture can often be diagnosed clinically by observing and examining the injured limb and noting swelling, bruising, pain, tenderness, and abnormal motion, its nature and extent are best revealed by an x-ray. When the injury first occurs, first-aid should include controlling movement at the break so that additional damage to the bone or nearby soft tissues is kept to a minimum. Arms or legs with suspected fractures can be splinted with wood or even with a pillow. Elevation helps to reduce swelling and bleeding.

The bonesetter's art is old, in some societies distinct from that of other healers. Many pretechnical communities practice bonesetting by traction, massage, manipulation, and immobilization, and achieve credible results. Hugh Owen Thomas, one of the founders of modern orthopaedics, came from a family of bonesetters who practiced their craft in Liverpool, England, during the early 1800s.

All forms of fracture treatment follow the basic rule that the broken pieces must be restored to their original positions (reduction) and prevented from moving (immobilization) until they have healed. This can be accomplished through:

- ❏ *Traction*, a sustained pull on the skin or through a metal pin placed in a bone. The pulling force is transmitted to the bone and by a gentle steady action normal length and alignment are accomplished.
- ❏ *Casting after repositioning,* which is achieved by manipulation under local or general anesthesia. A plaster or fiberglass cast is applied, and the joints above and below the fracture are immobilized. The most common type of bandage used is plaster of paris. Although introduced by the Dutch physician Anthonius Mathijson in 1852, it takes its name from the Montmartre district in Paris, from which the "plaster" was originally mined. Plaster of paris is anhydrous (without water) calcium sulfate produced by driving the water out of gypsum (the German word for cast is *gyps*) by heating. When a roll of plaster is dipped in water in preparation for applying a cast, it gives off heat.
- ❏ *A functional brace or cast brace* allows some control of movement of nearby joints and may be appropriate for some fractures of the long bones of the arms or legs.
- ❏ *Open reduction and internal fixation.* The orthopaedic surgeon may elect to operate on an unstable fracture and, after repositioning, rigidly hold the fracture fragments with any of a variety of screws, bolts, plates, or other internal splints. The metals from which these devices are made are usually stainless steel or titanium and chrome-cobalt or vitallium type alloys, which are sufficiently inert in the body so as not to initiate electrolytic activity that is detrimental to tissue healing. The advantages of internal fixation are that casts are not usually necessary and the treatment allows earlier movement of the limb, thereby avoiding the wasting and stiffness that accompany prolonged immobilization.
- ❏ *External fixation* involves the placement of pins or screws into the broken bone, above and below the site of the break. The bone fragments are then reduced and the pins or screws are connected to metal bars, from which a sta-

bilizing frame is constructed to hold the bones in their proper position for healing. After healing, the external fixation device is removed. This treatment is often used in open, comminuted, or complex fractures in which open reduction and internal fixation might cause further damage to the bone.

Because the aim of all fracture treatment is to maintain function, early exercise is usually encouraged. In each case, the treatment should be one that will restore the limb to full functional capacity as quickly and as safely as possible.

Deficient or defective healing of a fracture can occur for a number of reasons. The most disastrous complication is infection (osteomyelitis), which of course is more prevalent in open fractures and is a calculated risk when any operation exposing bone is undertaken. The use of meticulous cleansing techniques and an "antibiotic umbrella" help prevent this complication.

Bone is no different from any other body tissue in requiring an adequate blood supply for healing, which may be impaired when circulation is inadequate. It has been established among other things that smoking can delay bone healing. This can lead to nonunion of the fracture or even the formation of a false joint (pseudarthrosis) at the fracture site. Factors that can lead to slow union or nonunion include distraction (pulling apart) of bony fragments, interposition of soft tissues (particularly muscle), or loss of the fracture blood clot through an open wound. When reduction has been inadequate, shortening, angulation, or malrotation can occur at the fracture site and remain after healing. This condition is called "malunion" and, if severe enough, it may require surgical breaking and resetting of the bone.

Nonunions can be treated with grafts of fresh bone, usually taken from some location in the patient's body that has bone to spare (such as the pelvic wing) or from a bone bank, which provides bone cut into various sizes and segments, sterilized, and specially treated to avoid a foreign body response when used for transplantation. Bone or bone substitute are prepackaged as small pieces, chips, or even crystals, which make a thick slurry when added to a liquid. Current state of the art in the treatment of slow or nonunion of fractures also includes electrical stimulation with externally or internally applied magnetic fields to stimulate bone growth through the induction of a piezoelectric current.

Injuries that involve the bones and joints strike approximately one-quarter of the American population each year. On average, almost every American suffers some form of injury in each four-year period. These injuries result in nearly 20 million annual hospital days (the average length of stay is more than eight days, longer than for most other disorders). The cost associated with fracture treatment is estimated at $18 billion each year, almost half of which is attributable to hip fractures in the elderly. Approximately 35 million days are lost from work or school because of fractures. As would be expected, fractures in men are more frequent in the younger age group, whereas women predominate in the senior age category as the result of osteoporosis.

Preventing fractures is easier than treating them. As mentioned before, healthy bones are maintained by a diet that is adequate in proteins and minerals and by proper exercise. A lifestyle that avoids physical risks that may result in fracture may not be as thrilling as one that is characterized by hang gliding, mountain climbing, and motorcycling, but it is certainly safer.

Fractures suffered by earlier peoples and discovered through examination of their skeletons can be revealing. The so-called "taskmaster's fracture" (isolated fracture of the ulna bone of the forearm) has been seen frequently in the skeletal remains of Egyptian slaves. This evidence bears mute testimony to the fact that these slaves tried to ward off blows with their upraised arms. These days it is called a "nightstick fracture."

Typical fractures often associated with specific injuries are so named. The chauffeur's fracture (a broken bone in the forearm) was caused by a sudden and violent reversal of the crank used to start the old Model T Ford. Boxer's fracture is a break just below the knuckle, and hangman's fracture needs no explanation.

As you well know, bones are not the only musculoskeletal structures that are prone to injury. I have already alluded to the possibility of soft tissue injuries of the joints. Now it is time to read on and review these problems in detail.

FIRST AID FOR BROKEN BONES

The principle of first-aid treatment of broken bones is to minimize pain and prevent further injury. When a fracture is suspected:

1. Call a doctor immediately.

2. Do not move the injured part until it has been splinted. A suspected broken leg can be tied to the opposite well leg, or it can be bound onto a pillow or blanket, reinforced by two or three pieces of wood or rigid objects, such as a broomstick, mop handle, pole, baseball bat, rolled up magazine, or thick folded newspaper. The splint should be long enough to extend beyond the joints above and below the fracture. The splint should be padded with clothing or soft material, and the splint should be secured with strips of clothing or sheets in at least three places—beyond the joints on either side of the fracture and halfway between them.

If the skin is broken (open fracture):

1. Gently cut away or remove clothing from the injured extremity.

2. Place a sterile dressing or a clean handkerchief or towel over the wound and press firmly to control any bleeding.

3. Secure the pad with a strong bandage.

4. Call a doctor as soon as bleeding is under control.

5. Splint the part.

The treatment for suspected dislocations is the same as that for a closed fracture. Patients with suspected fractures of the spine (particularly the neck) should not be moved, even to a more comfortable position. They must be transported on a stretcher and brought immediately to the attention of a physician. Rigid support should be provided for the victim's back if possible. You must wait for adequate help, at least three and preferably four persons, to assist in transportation.

DOWN TO THE BONE ADVICE ON SPLINTS

1. Splints should be adequately padded between splint and skin, especially over places where there are bony protuberances.

2. Make sure the splint is not too tight. Complaints of numbness or inability to move the fingers or toes are indications that the splint is too tight and should be loosened.

3. Never test for a fracture before splinting by having the victim move the arm or leg, and *never* ask someone to walk on a leg with a suspected fracture. Remember that a limb can be moved even if it is broken.

QUESTIONS AND ANSWERS ABOUT FRACTURES

Q: Are plaster casts ever used for orthopaedic conditions other than fractures?

A: Plaster casts can be used to immobilize soft tissue injuries such as sprains and strains. They may also be applied after certain operations.

Q: Should any precautions be taken with a plaster cast?

A: The cast will feel warm while it is being applied. This is due to the chemical reaction that occurs during the setting of the plaster. It usually takes a day or so for the cast to completely dry, after which it will weigh considerably less than on initial application because of evaporation of water.

Swelling around an injury is common and may cause some pressure in the cast. Therefore, the part casted should be elevated as much as possible to reduce swelling. Ice in a plastic bag or an ice pack can also be applied to the cast to help keep swelling down. The cast should be kept uncovered until it is completely dry, and of course it should be protected from getting wet after this.

Needless to say, dirt and other foreign substances should be kept away from the inside of the cast. You should never push sharp objects inside the cast to relieve an itch. Your doctor should be advised if the cast becomes soft or cracked, or if your pain increases. Other signs that warn you to contact your physician immediately include (1) numbness, tingling, swelling, or blue discoloration in the fingers or toes; (2) burning in a cast (this usually indicates pressure or rubbing); (3) any evidence of secretions or drainage inside the cast (discoloration of the plaster or odor); (4) any fever or chills.

Q: Are fractures at or near a zone of bony growth (epiphyseal fractures) dangerous?

A: Some are, some are not. Growth arrest or abnormal growth sometimes complicate such fractures. The orthopaedic surgeon can determine this and sometimes can take measures to prevent it.

Q: Are there techniques of diagnosing fracture other than x-ray?

A: CT scanning is another method to determine the kind and degree of fracture. It is frequently used for fractures of the pelvis (particularly the hip socket) because it furnishes an excellent three-plane picture of the fracture, which a two-dimensional x-ray cannot provide. X-rays are sometimes used to "slice through a bone." This technique is called tomography and can reveal deep fracture or other pathology that a simple x-ray cannot. The technique of magnetic resonance imaging is best for the evaluation of soft tissue pathology.

Q: How long does it take for a plaster cast to fully dry?

A: That depends on the thickness of the cast as well as on humidity. However, the cast should be dry enough to handle in 10 minutes and should be thoroughly dry within 24 hours. Keeping the cast exposed to air during this time or using a heat lamp assists in drying. After the cast is dry, you should protect it by covering it with several well-secured plastic bags while showering or bathing. A hair dryer can be used to dry it if it gets damp.

5

Soft Tissue Injuries

Love is like a sprain, the second time it arrives more easily

Spanish Proverb

Sprains and contusions account for more than 40,000 days lost from school or work per year and almost 600,000 annual hospital discharges. Musculoskeletal soft tissue injuries—injuries involving muscles, tendons, ligaments, and so forth—are more common than fractures. All are caused by stress, which may be due either to a single overload or to chronic overuse.

Ligaments support joints and prevent them from dislocating. This tissue has an inherent elasticity, but it can stretch when stressed. Once stretched, a ligament tends to stay that way; it begins to tear when stretched over 6 percent of its resting length. Injury to a ligament is called a *sprain*. Sprains are classified according to severity: (a) grade 1, stretched ligament; (b) grade 2, partial tear; or (c) grade 3, complete tear.

The ligaments of the ankle and knee joints are put under considerable strain during athletic activity and therefore are most prone to this kind of damage. Stability of the outside of the ankle is less than that of the inside, and the joint is usually sprained by twisting the foot inward on the leg. Rotation injuries with the foot firmly planted are a common cause of knee sprains.

Sprains are usually treated with ice, rest while elevating the limb, and a supportive wrap. A plaster cast is used to immobilize the involved joint when more severe sprains occur, and complete rupture of a ligament may require surgical repair. Rehabilitation of the joint through appropriate exercises is important from the onset of treatment. After injury the muscles almost immediately begin to atrophy and weaken. For example, the muscles that straighten the knee can lose up to 25 percent of their strength within the first 48 hours after injury to this joint. Joint stiffness and calcium loss also complicate immobilization.

Direct blows to muscle cause a soft tissue injury called a *contusion*. Bleeding can occur if the blow is severe enough. This results in bruising of the skin and underlying soft tissues, accompanied by swelling. Deep muscular scarring, calcium deposition, or even bony formation secondary to muscle damage may occur.

Myositis ossificans is a condition characterized by the formation of bone in the soft tissues. It usually develops in muscle as the result of bleeding due to trauma. Such a mass of bone may restrict motion by obstruction or by decreasing elasticity in the involved muscle. A diagnosis of myositis ossificans is made

FIGURE 5-1 How a Ligament Heals

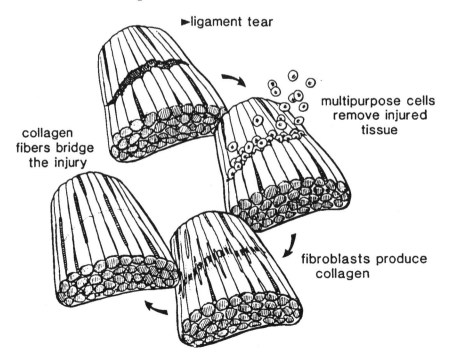

by history, physical examination, and an x-ray that reveals the bony deposit. Rest, elevation, and icing after trauma can prevent or control bleeding, decreasing the incidence of this condition. Once bone formation has developed, physical therapy is not advised because it can cause additional trauma and the development of still more unwanted bone. The bone can be excised if it is painful or disabling, but only after complete maturity of the bony mass is achieved. This may take three to six months. Premature removal could result in a recurrence that may be more extensive than the original mass.

Inflammation of a tendon is called *tendinitis* (*-itis* always means inflammation). Tennis elbow, swimmer's shoulder, and jumper's knee are examples of tendinitis at these joints that is caused by repetitive overuse. Treatment is directed at decreasing the inflammation with injections of anti-inflammatory drugs such as corticosteroids, or medications such as a nonsteroidal anti-inflammatory drug, icing, rest, and support. Because improper athletic techniques aggravated by poor sports mechanics or equipment and overtraining can frequently result in tendinitis, these causes should be sought out and remedied.

Tendons can also tear. The plantaris tendon (a vestigial structure in the calf) is frequently torn during sports such as tennis. A sudden snap is experienced in the calf. This is not a serious problem, only requiring rest for a brief period of time. A more critical condition is when the Achilles tendon tears. This is the strongest tendon in the body, but it can rupture when it is weakened and placed under undue stress. This often happens in the older weekend athlete, although it can occur in a trained athlete or a ballet dancer. This is a significant injury that may require surgery or at least prolonged casting for repair. More about the Achilles tendon will be discussed in Chapter 6 on fitness and bone.

You will remember that a muscle is connected to a bone or other tissue by tendon. Muscles are vulnerable at the site where they attach to tendons. Injury to the muscle-tendon unit is a *strain*, in which the tissue may be stretched or torn. Most strains occur in the lower extremities; for example, the hamstring injuries seen in football are usually strains. A muscle strain is treated much like its cousin, the sprain, with rest, ice, support, and protected motion.

Muscles and tendons that glide over bony prominences require a "buffer" between them and the bone to permit smooth gliding. A fluid-filled sac called a *bursa* does just this. Bursae are found around all joints (the knee alone has 14 of them). When they become irritated and inflamed because of repetitive use, the condition is called *bursitis*. Treatment is similar to that of other soft tissue injuries, but often also includes aspiration of inflammatory fluid from the bursa and injection of a corticosteroid to reduce inflammation. Chronic or recurrent bursitis, such as that of the olecranon (elbow tip) or shoulder may require surgical excision of the offending bursal sac. "Housemaid's knee" is bursitis of the bursa overlying the knee cap that occurs in people who scrub floors while on their knees. Modern stand-up mopping and waxing techniques have made this condition all but extinct. "Weaver's bottom" is an occupational ischial bursitis found in weavers who sit on hand stools or cross-legged on a firm floor while weaving.

Violent stress, chronic overuse, or aging can cause more serious injuries to soft tissues. The tendon complex supporting the shoulder is called the *rotator cuff*. Tears of this structure may result in chronic pain as well as an inability to lift the arm. This condition can be diagnosed by a special x-ray examination (arthrography) in which radiopaque dye injected into the shoulder is seen to leak out, or by an ultrasound or magnetic resonance imaging study. Surgery is often necessary. Diagnosis and repair can sometimes be accomplished through an *arthroscope*, which requires only a small incision and thus is followed by rapid healing.

Stress caused by chronic overuse can weaken bone to the point where a *stress fracture* can occur. This was initially seen in a metatarsal bone of the foot in draftees undergoing long marches. Hence it was called a "march fracture." It can occur as well in the heel bone, the tibia, or even the hip. Not readily apparent on an x-ray, a stress fracture might appear to be a sprain or strain and require a bone scan for diagnosis. Treatment is rest and immobilization, often with a plaster cast.

Needless to say, injuries to soft tissues can be prevented by proper athletic training, including appropriate warming up techniques. Overactivity is a set-up for soft tissue injury, especially of the "weekend type" and particularly when the athletic activity is age-inappropriate. Stretching and strengthening through isometric exercising are good techniques to keep the amateur athlete fit and functioning.

It is time now to put all these injuries in their proper perspective by seeing where they relate to sports activity.

QUESTIONS AND ANSWERS ABOUT SOFT TISSUE INJURIES

Q: What is lateral epicondylitis? Medial epicondylitis?

A: The *epicondyles* are the bumps at the sides of the elbow. The outside bump is the lateral epicondyle, the inside one the medial epicondyle. Lateral epicondylitis is called tennis elbow. It is due to an inflammation or tearing of the muscle tendons attached to the epicondyle. Medial epicondylitis is a similar condition at the inside of the elbow. It can be caused by a movement that twists the arm in, bending the wrist down, such as a golf swing. That is why this condition is often called golfer's or pitcher's elbow. Both lateral and medial epicondylitis are treated with cortisone injections, icing, rest, elbow straps, and NSAIDs. When unresponsive to this regimen, surgery may be necessary to release the offending tendon.

Q: Do tendon and ligament heal differently than bone?

A: Yes, soft tissue heals by multipurpose cells entering and cleaning up the injured area. These cells then express themselves as *fibroblasts* (cells that make soft tissue). The fibroblasts produce collagen, which is the framework for a new ligament or tendon. Eventually, the collagen is interwoven with that of the torn structure, the fibroblasts disappear, and a strong scar is formed (see Figure 5-1).

Bone also heals initially by multipurpose cells entering and cleaning up the injured area. These cells, however, become *osteoblasts*, which produce osteoid (bone collagen). This is mineralized, and new bone is created as the calcium and phosphorus crystals fill in the collagen framework. This is subsequently remodeled and eventually will heal without leaving a scar. Because no bone scar is formed, the healed bone should be as strong as it was before it was broken.

Q: What are some of the principles of recovery from a soft tissue injury?

A: Recovery from any injury begins the day that treatment is initiated. Even though an arm or leg is casted, muscle strength can be maintained, muscle wasting reduced, and circulation aided by isometric (tightening) exercises. Rehabilitation includes mobilizing joints through active or passive flexion and extension exercises, and sometimes the use of physical therapy treatments such as whirlpool, heat, massage, or ultrasound. Strengthening exercises and endurance training complete the program.

Q: Can we avoid losing muscle as we age?

A: Only by strength-training, which means contracting your muscles a few times against a heavy load. Even aerobic exercise (contracting your muscles many times with little or no resistance) does not prevent loss of muscle mass. Strength-training can be effective even if done for only 45 minutes twice a week.

Q: What kind of exercise lengthens life?

A: For a sedentary person, any regular exercise of moderate intensity. Especially helpful is resistance exercise (weight lifting) of large muscles such as the deltoids (shoulders) or quadriceps (thighs). This helps build muscle mass. The biggest jump in life expectancy is for people who go from doing nothing to being moderately active. And—it is never too late. Even if you are past 60, exercise will increase your life expectancy. Aerobic exercise increases HDL ("good") cholesterol and lowers blood pressure. In fact, if you have high blood pressure and you exercise, you will have a greater life expectancy than if you have normal blood pressure and do not exercise. Supervised balancing exercises like Tai Chi or some yoga postures, or even just standing on one leg, can help prevent falls in seniors and thus decrease the risk of hip fracture. It has been said that if exercise were a drug, it would be the most prescribed pill in the world.

6

Fitness and Bone

Sport, that wrinkled care derides. . .

John Milton L'Allegro—line 31

The Greek ethos of "sound mind, sound body" is wise to follow, but in pursuing a sound body through sport, realistic goals should be set and the athletic activity enjoyed by those participating in it. Some of you may be interested only in weight loss and general conditioning. Others may want special exercises to improve specific athletic activities. In any case, before embarking on any training program, you should see your doctor to make sure that the general condition of your body, especially your heart and lungs, is fit enough to undertake the exercise. In the case of children, parents and coaches should be reminded that winning is not everything. The enjoyment of the sport, conditioning of the body, and opportunity to play with a team are of prime importance.

PREVENTION OF INJURY

Almost 50 percent of American adults exercise regularly, and 10 percent of these suffer a sports-related accident each year. The cost of all of this, including hospital bills and lost work time, exceeds $39 billion a year. Proper conditioning can decrease the frequency and severity of many sports injuries. This involves the elements of endurance, strength, power, flexibility, and cardiovascular fitness. It includes the development of form, agility, and proper body mechanics. The specific training will depend on the athletic activity involved, but stretching and toning exercises can protect against ligamentous strain. Staying in shape during the off-season may require aerobic exercise at home.

STRETCHING EXERCISES

Here are some good stretching exercises that can be used as a general warmup for any sports activity, such as running, swimming, tennis, and so forth. They are also useful for cooling down after the activity.

1. Lie comfortably on your back with your knees bent. Take a deep breath and, exhaling, slide your right foot forward and back. Repeat with the left foot. Clench your fists tightly, then relax.

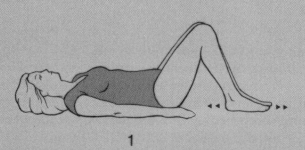

1

2. Lying on your back with the knees bent, breathe in and out deeply and slowly. Pull your shoulders up with every inhalation. Relax as you exhale.

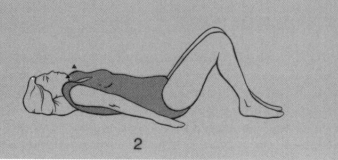

2

3. In the same position, turn your head as far to the right as possible. Return to the normal position and relax. Repeat the exercise turning your head to the left.

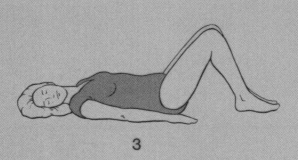

3

4. Lie on your back with your knees bent and pull both knees up to your chest. Lower them slowly to the floor.

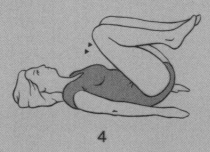

4

5. While kneeling with the weight resting on your hands and knees, arch your back, at the same time dropping your head.

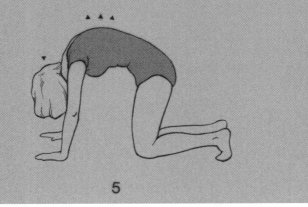

5

6. Still in the kneeling position, place your weight on your hands and knees. Gradually slide your arms forward until your forearms are resting on the floor. Move slowly back to the original position.

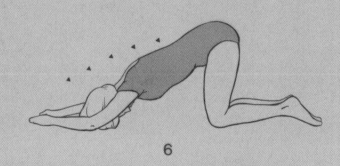

6

7. Lying on your back with your knees bent, place your hands on your abdomen and raise your head, your neck, and finally your shoulders from the floor. Return slowly to the starting position and repeat.

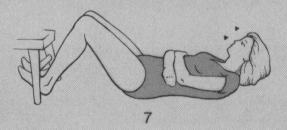

7

8. Lying on your back with your knees bent, first bring your left knee to your chest, then extend the left leg with toes pointed toward the ceiling. Keeping your left knee straight, lower the leg to the floor, then bring it back up to the flexed position. Repeat these movements with the opposite leg.

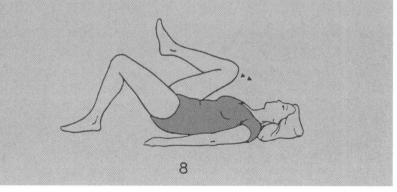

8

9. Still lying on your back with your knees bent, slide your left leg forward. With the knee locked, perform a straight leg lift, raising the leg as high as possible. Lower the leg slowly to the floor, slide it to the flexed position, and repeat with the opposite leg.

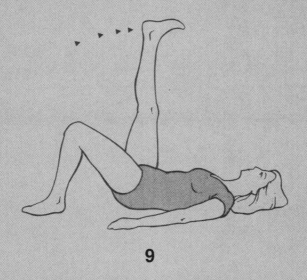

9

10. Standing with the heels together and the hands behind the back, bend slowly forward from the hips, moving down as far as you can.

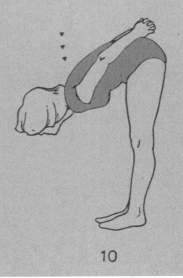

10

11. Stand an arm's length from a wall with both feet together, place your hands flat on the wall and keep your hips and knees straight. Using your hands and forearms for support, try to place your chest on the wall. You will feel a stretch in your heel cords. Straighten your arms and push your body back to the original position.

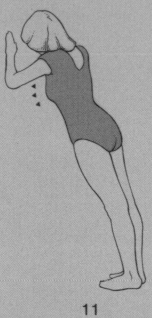

11

12. Standing with your heels together, take a deep breath. While you let it out slowly, bend forward from the waist, dropping your head, shoulders, and finally your hips. Do not force this exercise. You should feel some stretch in your back and the back of your legs. Relax and straighten up.

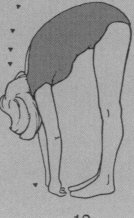

12

TABLE 6–1.   ENERGY EXPENDITURE OF SELECTED ACTIVITIES

Cal/min	Cal/hr	Activity
2.0–2.5	120–150	Strolling 1 miles/hour; light housework: polishing furniture
2.5–4.0	150–240	Walking at 2 miles/hour; golf using power cart
4–5	240–300	Walking at 3 miles/hour; golf pulling cart, cleaning windows, mopping floors, vacuuming
5–6	300–360	Walking 3.5 miles/hour; golf carrying clubs, doubles tennis, table tennis
6–7	360–420	Walking 4 miles/hour; ice or roller skating
7–8	420–480	Walking 5 miles/hour; singles tennis
8–10	480–600	Jogging 5 miles/hour; paddleball, downhill skiing
10–11	600–660	Running 5.5 miles/hour; squash or handball
11	660	Running 6–8 miles/hour

EVALUATE YOURSELF

Here is a set of standards with which to evaluate yourself. They are indicators of overall physical fitness, not endurance alone. The exercises are described on the next page. Figures in parentheses are for men 40 years or older.

Remember to take it easy at the outset of this program. Start at a level you can handle and gradually increase.

		NUMBER OF REPETITIONS				
EXERCISE	PERFORM-ANCE TIME	UNSAT	SAT	GOOD	EXCEL-LENT	OUT-STANDING
STRETCHER	2 min	0–22	23–24	25–26	27–29	30 & above
		(0–19)	(20–22)	(23–24)	(25–26)	(27 & above)
SIT-UPS	60 sec	0–19	20–24	25–29	30–35	36 & above
		(0–15)	(16–20)	(21–24)	(25–29)	(30 & above)
PUSH-UPS	60 sec	1–14	15–16	17–19	20–24	25 & above
		(1–12)	(13–14)	(15–17)	(18–20)	(21 & above)
SUSTAINED JUMPING	60 sec	0–5	6–10	11–16	17–25	26 & above
		(0–4)	(5–8)	(9–14)	(15–20)	(21 & above)
STATIONARY RUN	6 min	0–350	351–410	411–525	526–650	651 & above
		(0–300)	(301–375)	(376–450)	(451–550)	(551 & above)

FIVE EXERCISES TO BUILD PHYSICAL ENDURANCE

Although muscular strength can be built through an isometric program, endurance requires both muscular and cardiovascular activity. In order to increase endurance, you must extend yourself by increasing either the speed of the exercise or its duration. Eleven minutes are required to perform the five exercises described here. They should be done at least every other day and if possible daily.

1. *Stretcher*—2 minutes. Keeping your feet apart, touch outside the left foot, between the feet and outside the right foot, with both hands. Come to an upright position and circle bend as far as possible. This is one full count. Repeat exercise as many times as possible within the two-minute period.

2. *Push-ups*—1 minute. Do push-ups, keeping your legs straight. Repeat as many as possible within the one minute period.

3. *Sit-ups*—1 minute. Do sit-ups with your knees bent to protect your back. Perform as many as possible within the one minute period.

4. *Sustained jump*—1 minute. Determine the highest point you can jump and reach when fully stretched and mark it on a wall. See how many times you can come close to this mark in one minute.

5. *Stationary run*—6 minutes. Running in place, bring the feet up in front at least five inches off the floor. Each time your right foot hits the floor is one count. After 100 full counts, do 10 stride jumps. These will prevent cramping in your legs. Continue this exercise for six minutes.

You should begin any athletic activity gradually. Stretching is especially important to avoid strain. The heel cords, hamstrings, and quadriceps (front of the thigh) muscles should be given special attention. Because tissues stretch better when warm, stretching is best performed after five minutes of slow walking. Stretching should be slow and gradual through full movement, holding the maximum stretched position for 20 to 30 seconds before relaxing. No pain should be felt. As important as warming up before exercise is cooling off afterward. Rather than simply standing still or lying down after vigorous activity, it is better to walk around for a few minutes and also to do some mild stretching exercises.

A CATALOG OF SPORTS INJURIES

Injuries to muscles, such as strains and sprains, are covered in Chapter 5. Muscle cramps can occur during or after exercise.

They are usually due to the accumulation of waste products (lactic acid) and most often affect the muscles of the legs. Proper warming up can often prevent cramping, as can maintaining adequate fluid intake. It is never appropriate for an athlete to try to run through pain. When cramps occur at night after exercise, relief can be obtained through icing and massage.

Muscular bruising is common to many sports. Roller blade skating leads the list for injury to the weekend athlete. Treatment is designed to avoid complications and return the athlete to full activity as soon as possible. Icing and rest will control swelling and pain. An elastic compression dressing may be necessary. Activities should be resumed only after complete recovery.

INJURIES OF THE UPPER EXTREMITY

The Shoulder

The shoulder is a ball and socket joint that sacrifices stability for range of motion. The flexibility of the shoulder is the greatest of any joint in the body. This places a great deal of stress on the shoulder capsule and the muscles that stabilize the shoulder and contribute to the tendinous rotator cuff that encloses this joint. Throwing motions may lead to overuse injury, particularly the common movement of over-arm throwing. Such damage may be a simple irritation of the tendon or a bursitis, or a more complicated tear (rupture) of the rotator cuff. The soft tissues of the shoulder often respond to injury by calcifying. Shoulder pain is present and may radiate down the arm or up the neck. The shoulder is tender to palpation (pressure). Stiffness with decreased range of motion may be seen. These findings frequently show up in swimmers because of the length and intensity of their training regimens.

Treatment of rotator cuff irritation or inflammation is usually conservative. It includes rest, ice, and avoiding the offending activity. Oral anti-inflammatory agents are prescribed and sometimes local injections of steroid may be helpful. Repetitive injections should be avoided, however, as tendon rupture has occurred after indiscriminate use of injections. For this reason, vigorous exercise of the shoulder should not be allowed following injections. Proper throwing and correct swimming mechanics should be taught.

Surgical repair may be necessary for a complete rotator cuff rupture. Diagnosis (and sometimes treatment) of such an injury can often be accomplished with an arthroscopy of the shoulder. Arthroscopic procedures involve distending the joint with fluid and introducing a slender fiberoptic light source arthroscope through a small incision (portal). Attached to the scope is a miniature video camera so the interior of the joint can be viewed and projected onto a color television monitor. Instrumentation is accomplished by localizing with triangulation through other portals. Procedures are carried out while the joint is constantly being filled and flushed with fluid. A variety of specialized scissors, angled cutters, electric grinders, graspers, and other instruments enable the skilled operator to accomplish almost any surgical task without opening the joint. Other shoulder conditions, such as impingement and pinching of the soft tissue structures of the shoulder, can also be treated with arthroscopic surgery.

"Little league shoulder" is an irritation of the bony growth zone (epiphysis) of children who participate in little league baseball. This condition is due to traction of the muscles about the shoulder resulting in irritation of the growth zone of the upper humerus. X-rays may reveal bony reaction to the trauma. The disorder is treated with rest and leaves no residuals.

"Shoulder pointer" is an injury to the point of the shoulder by a direct blow. The muscles as well as the joint at the end of the clavicle (collarbone) at the shoulder are injured. Rest, ice, and a nonsteroidal anti-inflammatory drug usually heal the damage in short order.

"Shoulder separation" usually refers to a partial or complete dislocation of the clavicle where it joins the shoulder at the *acromioclavicular joint*. Minor injuries can be treated with rest, but a complete separation in the dominant shoulder of an athlete whose sport requires throwing (commonly a football quarterback) will often require surgical repair. However, except for a bump on the shoulder, most individuals with complete dislocation at this joint have no pain or serious disability. Treating the dislocation in a sling for three to six weeks and then leaving it alone is acceptable therapy. If the deformity is too unsightly, a simple operation to remove a small portion of the clavicle at the shoulder can be performed at a later date.

Most shoulder dislocations occur from falls on the out-stretched arm, when the shoulder joint is rotated up and back. The ball portion of the ball and socket joint is dislocated anteri-orly (in front). Treatment consists of reducing the dislocation. This should be done as soon as possible because muscle spasm can make reduction difficult, particularly in a robust athlete. Putting the shoulder back into place can often be accomplished without a general anesthetic, if the patient can relax and permit the doctor to pull and rotate the shoulder. Occasionally an anes-thetic is needed to obtain full relaxation. After reduction, the arm should be restrained for at least three weeks. A sling can be used for the last portion of this immobilization. At night, the sleeve should be pinned to the pajama body to prevent redislo-cating the shoulder when asleep. After three weeks, mobiliza-tion to prevent permanent stiffness is begun with pendulum exercises, which eliminate the need to lift the arm against gravity. General strengthening exercises are then started, and the athlete gradually returns to his activity.

For recurrent dislocations of the shoulder, immobilization will not prevent redislocation. After reduction, the shoulder should be held in a sling until pain and spasm are gone. The joint should be examined for any nerve damage that may have occured at the time of dislocation. A tether may be worn during activity to restrict the up and out motion that dislocates the shoulder. Surgery may eventually be necessary to tighten up the shoulder and block further dislocation.

The so-called "slipping shoulder" is due to weakness and stretching of the shoulder capsule, which permits the joint to slip but not fully dislocate. This causes pain, weakness, and apprehension, particularly when the arm is rotated up and out. If appropriate exercises fail, a surgical procedure is available to tighten the stretched structures and restore stability to the shoulder.

Stretching of the nerves that enter the arm from the neck (the brachial plexus) is unique to the sport of American football. Such an injury is called a "stinger" or "burner." It results from a sudden and violent depression of the shoulder with stretching of the neck to the opposite side. This often occurs when ramming the head in tackling or blocking. The stinger is characterized by sudden pain in the neck that can radiate to the hand. The pain is burning in nature, and transient weakness may occur. Treatment is usually unnecessary. However, if symptoms persist for more than a few minutes, a more serious injury, even a fracture in the neck, should be ruled out before allowing the athlete to return to play.

The Elbow

"Little league elbow" is caused by the repetitive act of throwing, particularly in pitchers, which places great stress on the elbow. Children, whose bony structures are immature, are subject to having chips of bone torn off (avulsion fractures), developing an inflammation of the growing parts of the bone (osteochondritis), having loose cartilage in the joint (joint mice), and a variety of other bony and soft tissue injuries. The elbow is painful and stiff. Symptoms may be either of acute onset or chronic in nature. Examination reveals a restricted range of motion and an x-ray may show the bony injury and effusion (fluid) in the joint. For the little leaguer, treatment is usually conservative, consisting of rest and eliminating the offending activity. Some of these injuries require months of inactivity in order to heal. In the case of a loose body, surgical removal can be performed, usually through an arthroscope.

The best treatment for little league elbow is prevention. In order to protect the elbow, no more than five to six innings of baseball should be pitched each week, and at least four to five days off should be allowed between games.

"Tennis elbow" is an irritation-inflammation of the lateral epicondyle (outer protuberance) of the elbow caused by strain and minor tearing of the tendon attaching to the bone at that point. This tendon is called the *common extensor-supinator tendon* because it attaches to muscles that extend (bend back) and supinate (rotate the palm up) the wrist. An improper backhand stroke is always the cause of tennis elbow in tennis players. Evert-Lloyd, Borg, Connors, and others, in popularizing the two-handed backhand, have done much to decrease the incidence of tennis elbow. However, this condition occurs far more frequently in anyone engaging in any activity that requires twisting the wrist with the elbow straight. Factory workers, mechanics, and homemakers are prone to this annoying injury.

Treatment is to first stop, or at least modify, the offending activity. Tennis players should play their backhand with the elbow and wrist rigid. The racquet should be large and made of metal alloy or other springy composite material designed to absorb stress on contact with the ball. Increasing the grip size can sometimes help. A strap tightly wrapped just below the elbow will redirect the force generated by the muscle giving some relief during play. Icing and aspirin or other NSAIDs are prescribed, and local injections of steroids will usually provide relief. Acupuncture sometimes helps. Forearm strengthening exercises such as wrist curls can prevent recurrences. Resistant cases require surgery to release the tendon at its origin.

Swelling of the bursa over the point of the elbow can occur due to a single trauma or repeated pressure. Aspiration and icing give relief. For recurrent or chronic swelling the bursa may have to be removed surgically.

The Hand

Sports injuries to the hand, including mallet (baseball) finger and jammed finger, as well as digit dislocations will be considered in Chapter 13 on the hand.

REHABILITATION EXERCISES FOR TENNIS ELBOW

These elbow exercises can be performed using no weight or a set of dumbbells or other weights, which can be increased a pound at a time from 3 to 8 pounds. Each of the four steps increases in difficulty. The player moves up only after mastering the preceding step.

Step 1. Firmly grip a 3 pound dumbbell in the symptomatic hand and then place the forearm palm down on a firm surface with the wrist positioned at the edge so that the hand gripping the dumbbell hangs free. Bend the wrist upward and toward the thumb as far as possible. Hold this position for four seconds, then return to the starting position and rest for three seconds. Repeat this ten times, gradually increasing to 15 times.

Step 2. Hold the dumbbell as in Step 1, this time with the palm up. Bend the wrist upward toward the ceiling as far as possible. Hold this position as before, rest, and repeat.

Step 3. Again, holding the dumbbell as in Step 1 with the palm down, rotate the wrist straight up toward the ceiling as far as possible. Hold, rest, and repeat as above.

Step 4. Beginning with the palm down, rotate the forearm 180 degrees, bringing the palm upward and the dumbbell to horizontal. This motion should take about four seconds. Repeat ten times, building up to 15 times.

Endurance will have been developed when all of these exercises can be easily performed, using a 3 to 8 pound weight 15 times. Routines can be repeated but this time they should be performed quickly with no rest between repetitions.

"Bowler's thumb" is a painful irritation and swelling of a nerve (neuroma) where the thumb grips the bowling ball. Pain and tenderness are present, and there may be numbness in the thumb. Rest, ice, and changing the bowling grip or ball as well as using an available protective device can prevent this condition.

INJURIES OF THE LOWER EXTREMITY

Ligamentous injuries and injuries to the cartilages of the knee are covered in chapter 11, and sprains and injuries to the ankle and foot are discussed in Chapter 12. A common football (and soccer) injury is a contusion to the brim of the pelvis called a "hip pointer." A large accumulation of blood (hematoma) can develop. This injury can be very painful. Rest and ice are used for the initial pain. Activity is permitted as tolerated, and a protective pad can be worn over the pelvis to prevent further injury.

"Turf toe" is a condition of jamming or forced hyperextension (bending up) of the big toe. This can result in a swollen, stiff, tender, inflamed (red) joint. Soft-soled shoes and artificial turf increase vulnerability to this injury. Treatment involves "RICE" therapy: **R**estricting motion by taping the toe, **I**cing, applying a **C**ompression dressing, and **E**levation. Rehabilitation includes exercises, whirlpool, and ultrasound treatments. Athletes who are prone to turf toe should wear stiff-soled shoes during play.

Gymnasts, football linemen, and ballet dancers must repeatedly bend and stress the front of their ankles while playing or performing. This impingement on the ankle can cause a pressure reaction with a build-up of excess bone that sometimes has to be removed surgically.

MISCELLANEOUS PROBLEMS

Young athletes often *avulse* or pull bone away at muscle origins. This is due to underconditioning and violent stretching during activity. Such trauma is most frequent about the shoulders and hips. The injury causes sudden pain, and an x-ray usually reveals the fragment of bone that has been pulled off, resulting in an *avulsion fracture*. Treatment will depend on what area has been damaged. A professional athlete may require an operation to reattach the avulsed tendon, but the recreational sportsman is often treated conservatively with rest until healing has occurred.

Any athlete with a neck injury should not be moved until an evaluation on the field has been performed. This is important because moving a person who has a fracture or dislocation of the neck can cause permanent damage to the spinal cord with resultant paralysis. Head ramming tackles are illegal in high school and college football for this reason. In fact, injury to the head and neck is the most frequent catastrophic sports injury; fatalities in football from 1973 to 1983 exceeded deaths in all other competitive sports combined. From 1931 to 1986 at least 819 deaths were directly attributed to high school and college football. In addition, there were cases of permanent quadriplegia (four limb paralysis) from spinal cord trauma. A biomechanical engineer once calculated that if two 200-pound football players ran into each other head-on it would take a helmet six feet thick (sic!) to fully absorb the shock.

Other sports with a high inherent risk of head and spine injury include boxing, ice hockey, horseback riding (as with Christopher Reeve's broken neck), wrestling, rugby, and gymnastics. The trampoline was discontinued as a gymnastic event because of an unacceptable rate of serious injury; the vault event recently led to quadriplegia in an elite female teenaged U.S. gymnast and may also be eliminated. When a broken neck is suspected, a collar can be used to immobilize the neck and the athlete moved on a stretcher.

The loose-jointed athlete is at higher risk for injuries to the ligaments, whereas the player who has tight joints is more vulnerable to muscular injuries. Loose jointedness affects girls more than boys, and it is often familial. Joints usually tighten up during late adolescence. Prior to this time the athlete is vulnerable to injury, especially to the joints of the knees and ankles. Loose-jointed athletes need strengthening exercises to avoid ligament injury and strain. Tight-jointed athletes require stretching exercises to increase flexibility.

THE YOUNGER ATHLETE

Growing bodies require different conditioning than those that are already mature. There is notable and increasing popularity of sports among young people. Statistics tell us that over 50 percent of boys and 30 percent of girls between the ages of 9 and 17 participate in an organized sports program some time during the year. The National Federation of State High School Associations reports that more than half of all middle schools and junior high schools have competitive interscholastic athletic programs, and 5.2 million high school students participate in approximately 30 different types of competitive sports. The sports with the greatest number of participants during the past season were football (942,279), basketball (916,653—combined total for boys and girls), and track-and-field (757,703 for both sexes).

Young athletes are significantly different from adults. Because their skeletons are still growing, they are more susceptible to injury, particularly during growth spurts. There are also significant differences between individual children as the result of variations in body fat and muscle. Coaches bear the prime responsibility for spotting injuries and seeing that they are treated promptly and adequately. Coaches and parents share a duty to create a psychological attitude that encourages cooperation and self-sufficiency, learning to deal with defeat as well as success.

Fortunately, most sports injuries in young people are sprains, strains, and contusions. These are easily treated with rest, icing, and compression wrapping. Spinal cord injuries can be minimized by proper conditioning exercises that strengthen the neck and back. Fractures are rare, except for stress fractures, which are most frequently seen in the tibia, the fibula, and the foot.

In examining a child it is wise to remember that pain may be referred elsewhere from the point of injury. For example, pain along the inside of the knee can actually be caused by an injury of the hip.

Today's young women are able to train and compete on a level with their male counterparts. There may be some differences in athletic performance that correlate with gender, but injuries more often than not are related to the sport rather than the sex of the participant.

RUNNING INJURY

A 185 pound, 5 foot 10 1/2 inch tall runner whose running stride is one yard long will absorb approximately 350,000 pounds of stress on his feet for each mile he runs. It is not surprising that one of every two runners will at some time sustain an injury that will prevent running. In experienced runners, such injuries are usually related to overuse, such as increasing mileage too quickly. In beginning runners, they are most often due to being out of shape or running too much or too soon on hard surfaces in poor shoes.

Almost a third of running injuries occur at the knee. Strain to the heel cords are the second most common site of injury. Leg cramps due to "shin splints" fall third, and foot problems are last.

Pain is nature's way of indicating that something is wrong, and a runner should never try to "run through" or "run out" an injury. Doing so may convert a minor problem to a major one. There is no gain to pain here.

Novice or beginning runners may suffer muscle soreness or strain, low back pain, or knee pain secondary to chondromalacia (softening of the articular cartilage of the kneecap) because of improper training technique or unsuitable shoes. Overuse syndromes are seen when a runner progresses too rapidly from one level of training to another, increasing his speed and distance without allowing his body to slowly and comfortably adapt to a higher stress level. The long-distance runner can sustain serious muscle injury and, although this book focuses on orthopaedic problems, it should be mentioned that long-distance runners are also vulnerable to cold or heat injury during competition.

Factors Contributing to Running Injury

Training errors, including over-intensive workouts and rapid increase in mileage, simply overtax the body's ability to adapt to new stress levels. Inadequate warmup contributes to this problem.

Running on a springy level surface, such as a cinder track, dirt path, or grass, is ideal. However, many people run on hard surfaces, such as concrete or asphalt. This exaggerates the shock transmitted from the feet through the knees to the hips and back. A banked surface, such as the shoulder of a road, places unequal weight and stress on the legs. Running uphill produces tension on the heel cords and muscles of the low back, and downhill running increases impact on the heel. Excessive strain on the feet, such as that placed on the outer heel, can create an imbalance that is transmitted upward, causing pain in the knee.

Distance walking, particularly race walking, is an excellent aerobic exercise, offering many of the advantages of running without most of the risks of running injury. The benefits of brisk walking are numerous: proper body weight and muscle tone are maintained (especially in the buttocks, thighs, and hips). Walking helps keep the appetite stable and burns calories and body fat; it relieves anxiety; and because walking increases blood flow to the brain, it stimulates creative thinking patterns. If you are a walker, you will be familiar with the rhythmic, almost meditative qualities engendered by this exercise. Approximately one-fifth of all U.S. walkers walk nearly 3 miles a day, or more than 1,000 miles a year. Before starting such a program, you should consult your doctor about planning a workout that is tailored to your ability and needs. You should wear comfortable clothing and well-cushioned shoes that offer good shock absorption and lateral support. Remember to warm up with some stretching exercises and swing your arms back and forth to get your circulation going.

You can monitor your heart rate during your walk. Just subtract your age from 220. Now multiply that number by both 0.6 and 0.8 to determine your target pulse rate range. A healthy 50-year-old should maintain a pulse rate between 102 and 136 beats a minute for maximum conditioning. Walking 15 to 30 minutes a day, three days a week, at 60 percent maximum heart rate is considered light walking; 45 minutes a day, five days a week at 70 percent maximum is active walking; and one hour a day, five days a week at 80 percent maximum is power walking. If you prefer to exercise with others, walking is your sport. You can even join a walking club. It is great fun to walk and talk and if you can do this without trouble breathing, you are walking at a proper pace. Finally, if you are shy of the elements you can find a nearby mall and "mall walk" in its climate-controlled confines. Now let's quicken our stride a bit and get back to running.

A runner can place two to six times his body weight on the supporting foot. Each foot strikes the ground 50 to 60 times a minute (1,000 to 2,000 times per mile), thus placing considerable strain on the running shoe (which incidentally loses up to 30 percent of its ability to absorb shock after 500 miles of use), which is then transmitted directly to the leg and back. Most runners run with a heel-toe gait, making the heel very vulnerable at heel strike. During running, the foot rotates and the knee flexes and then straightens. The pelvis also rotates to keep the body level. Ideally, a runner should maintain an upright posture with the upper body and arms relaxed, and the elbows bent to approximately 90 degrees with the hands held loosely opened. Flexing the elbows further and clenching the fists during running can cause tension pain in the shoulders. Swinging the arms across the body accentuates the rotation of the pelvis and may cause muscular strain and pain.

Biomechanical imbalance in the knees, ankles, and feet can set the stage for running injuries. Running can be very hard on your knees if you have either bowlegs or knock-knees. The runner should suspect such an imbalance if he notes calluses, blisters, or any deformation of the foot, such as bunions, flat foot, or excessive height of the long arch. You are bowlegged if when you stand with your ankles together your knees do not touch. You have knock-knees if you can stand with your knees touching but your ankles cannot come together.

A runner's shoes bear testimony to faulty body mechanics or poor running habits. Wear in the forefoot area means that the runner is running on his toes. Wear on the outside of the heel, if severe, may indicate bowlegs causing knee pain. The running shoe should have a flexible sole with a firm long arch support, a heel that is outflared for added stability, and a stiff heel counter with a padded extension. The tongue should be well cushioned and the toe box high and rounded. The sole should be studded and the last straight. The midsole must be flexible (Figure 6-2). Certain shoe modifications are possible to treat or prevent injury; for example, heels can be split and wedged and foam rubber padding inserted in the sole to pad the metatarsal heads.

Use is not abuse! The key concept here is *gradual conditioning*. Runners must "warm up" prior to running with ham-

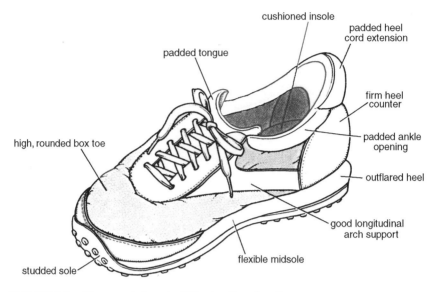

FIGURE 6-2   Characteristics of a Winning Running Shoe

string, heel cord, and back stretching. Equally important is a cooling down period with similar exercises after each run. Running time and mileage should be increased gradually, and running should be practiced on a regular basis. Any pain experienced is a signal to stop running.

A running injury that does not respond to a reasonable period of rest, icing, and aspirin should be brought to the attention of a doctor. The physician will take a history, which will focus on running habits, past history of deformity or injury, and any acquired conditions. The physical examination will localize the site of injury and determine the presence of any biomechanical problems that may contribute to the pain, such as leg length discrepancy, foot deformity, knock-knee, or bowleg.

X-rays will be taken to evaluate joints and rule out stress fracture. Special examinations such as bone scans and arthroscopy may be indicated in unusual cases. It has been noted that orchestra conductors and concert musicians seem to live longer than joggers and runners. Eugene Ormandy died at age 85, Efrem Zimbalist at 95. Joggers appear not to live so long. John B. Kelly, Jr. (U.S. Olympic Committee) died "clad in his running clothes" at age 58, and James Fixx at 51. Other long-lived conductors and musicians include Karl Boehm, 86; Arthur Fiedler, 86; Adrian Bouh, 100; Arturo Toscanini, 90; Richard

Strauss, 86; Leopold Stokowski, 96; Eubie Blake, 100; and Arthur Rubinstein, 94. This could be related to the benefit to the heart from exercising the arms aerobically, such as waving a baton on a podium. This jogging with the arms has been termed *jarming*.

THE INJURIES

The Knees

Chondromalacia syndrome is so common that it is referred to as "runner's knee." Some people's kneecaps are situated either higher or lower than normal. This contributes to unusual wear during bending and straightening the joint, which in turn causes irritation of the articular cartilage of the patella (kneecap). Excessive knock-knee or bowleg displaces the patella from its groove in the femur at the knee, causing unusual wear. The initial pain is aching after running a distance. It is frequently experienced by a runner who has just increased his mileage, and is often more severe after sitting for a prolonged period of time. In fact, stiffness of the knee after sitting, for an obvious reason called "theater knee," may be the symptom that first brings the runner to his doctor.

Treatment consists of rest, application of ice, vitamin C, and an anti-inflammatory drug such as aspirin. After several days, moist heat is substituted for the ice. Strain to the patella must be avoided, such as that incurred with stair-climbing, prolonged sitting, or kneeling. After the acute pain is gone, quadriceps strengthening exercises are initiated. A variety of knee braces and supports are available for this condition. Some of the most popular include straps that are placed below the kneecap and horseshoe-shaped patellar-conforming knee sleeves. Orthotic shoe devices may aid in realigning the knee. Steroid injection into the joint is seldom necessary. Surgery is rarely performed but, when indicated, shaving of the patella can be accomplished arthroscopically.

Treatment of inflammation of tendons about the knee, such as that along the lateral (outside) aspect of this joint or in the back of the knee, includes ice-friction massage (vigorously rubbing the area with ice until it is numb), rest, and anti-inflammatory medication. Inflammation of the tendon of the patella (jumper's knee) is treated in a similar manner.

The Lower Leg and Foot

"Shin splints" is an irritation of the tendons in the front-inside of the lower leg. This overuse syndrome usually develops in poorly conditioned athletes. It can also be caused by wearing an improper running shoe. A *tendinitis* occurs and should be treated by rest, icing, and elastic support. "Shin splints" can be prevented by running on a soft, level surface with proper shoes that prevent hyperpronation (excessive flattening) and rotation of the foot. An arch support may be necessary to accomplish this.

With persistent pain, an x-ray and sometimes a bone scan are necessary to rule out a stress fracture of the tibia. The best way to prevent stress fracture is to avoid overuse by scheduling loading and nonloading activities on alternate days. For example, alternate a day of running with a day of biking or swimming or simply resting. Stress fractures can also occur in the navicular bone of the foot. This is a particularly worrisome injury, sometimes even requiring surgery. It is common in gymnasts, and basketball player Bill Walton suffered from such a fracture for years.

Heel cord or Achilles tendinitis is a painful inflammation of the Achilles tendon (Figure 6-3). This injury is seen frequently in basketball players. The amount of body contact allowed in basketball has increased, players are larger, and more athletes are playing basketball. As a result, contact injuries such as contusions, sprains (such as the ankle sprain Scottie Pippen suffered during the 1997 Chicago Bulls playoff season), and stress fractures have increased.

This type of tendinitis is often caused by excessive tightness of the heel cords, thus the need for pre-running heel cord stretching. Running shoes that have rigid soles predispose to the condition, as does running up or down hills. Repetitive stress causes a burning pain that is worse during the early part of a run, improves during the run, then recurs afterwards. Tenderness of the heel cord is experienced, and swelling may be present. Treatment includes rest and icing followed by gentle stretching. Oral anti-inflammatory medication is helpful, and a

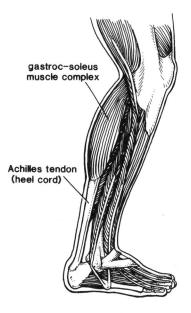

FIGURE 6-3   The Vulnerable Achilles Tendon

modification of running habits to avoid those practices that cause or aggravate Achilles tendinitis is necessary. Modification of the running shoe to include a flexible sole and a heel wedge and lift may relax the Achilles tendon at heel strike. Chronic Achilles tendinitis may require surgical correction.

The vulnerability of the heel cord was immortalized in Greek mythology, when Thetis, Achilles' mother, dipped him in the River Styx at birth intending to make him invulnerable. However, she held him by the heel and the water failed to cover Achilles' heel tendon. He was later slain by an arrow shot by Paris, and guided by Apollo, which struck him in the heel, his only weak point. The ancient Greeks were no doubt familiar with Achilles tendinitis as they ran a great deal. The Olympic games originated in Greece. One famous run was the 40 kilometer (approximately 25 miles) from Marathon to Athens in 490 B.C. to proclaim victory over the Persians. Competitive races in ancient Greece were usually no longer than three miles. However, to honor the original endurance champion, the first modern marathon held at the 1896 Athens Games followed its famous 24 mile path. The distance of the race varied until the 1908 games in London. The Queen requested that the route be altered so she could watch it from her window at the palace. The race covered 26 miles. The present marathon distance has been fixed at 26.2 miles, and my marathoner friends tell me it is that last 0.2 mile that does you in!

Bursitis about the heel can be treated by a local steroid injection. Heel bruise is caused by stepping on something irregular, like a pebble. A rigid plastic heel cup that shapes and supports the heel pad can offer definitive relief and prevent repeated injury.

Heel spurs are the most common cause of heel pain in runners. The pain is actually due to an irritation of the thick tissue, or *fascia*, that attaches at the heel spur. An inflammation of this tissue causes pain on heel strike. A loose, poorly fitting heel counter does not support the fat pad of the heel, permitting increased transmission of impact to the bone. Other biomechanical problems may be associated with this condition, such as severe flat foot. Rest, ice, heel pads, and a local injection of steroid are usually successful in curing the inflammation. Surgery is seldom indicated.

Painful bony prominences with overlying bursae are sometimes seen about the heel. Ice followed by warm soaks, oral anti-inflammatory medications, and appropriate padding is the treatment of choice.

Stress fractures of the metatarsal shafts can also occur, particularly in novice runners. Immobilization with either a cast or strapping is necessary, and healing usually occurs in four to six weeks.

Back and Hip Pain

Abnormal pelvic tilt during running can cause inflammation of a bursa over the side of the hip (greater trochanteric area) as well as the pelvic bone upon which we sit (the ischium). Rest and ice are usually all that is necessary for treatment, but local injection of steroid may be helpful. A leg length discrepancy should be looked for and treated with an appropriate shoe lift. Straining or partial tearing of muscles about the pelvis and leg is not uncommon, particularly in the hamstring muscles in the back of the thigh, and especially in adolescents doing speed work or uphill running. Treatment again is with ice and rest; weight-bearing activity should be curtailed.

Pain down the leg originating in the back may be due to a slipped lumbar disc. Often there is a history of a previous back problem. The athlete should stop running and the condition should be investigated with specialized tests such as electromyography, CT scanning, MRI imaging, and even myelography. Treatment consists of rest, traction, appropriate physical therapy, anti-inflammatory medication, and in some instances disc injections or surgery.

Irritation of the pubic joint in the front of the pelvis may result from repeated rotational pelvic strain during running, which produces a shearing force at this joint, the pubic symphysis. Gentle stretching exercises of the adductor muscles on the inside of the thigh may help prevent such injury; rest and heat are the treatment when it occurs.

Fractures due to muscle pull about the pelvis are sometimes seen. Prolonged rest for as long as several months may be necessary until symptoms abate, after which the runner can gradually return to his routine.

The treatment of running injuries is essentially conservative. These problems all require rest and distance reduction. A change in training is necessary. Ice for the acute pain followed by moist heat is usually indicated. Stretching exercises can often speed recovery and prevent reinjury. It cannot be emphasized enough that every person contemplating a running program should first have a physical examination. A previously sedentary individual should begin his running program slowly, first by walking on a soft, level surface and then by alternate jogging and walking. The running program should be individualized.

We cannot all be athletes, even amateur ones, yet exercise is important for physical conditioning. We all stand, we all should walk. The way we stand and walk—and sit as well—contributes to our skeletal alignment, our feeling of well-being, and the continued health of our bones and joints. This is where posture is important and this is what we will talk about next.

QUESTIONS AND ANSWERS ABOUT SPORTS INJURIES

Q: Are there doctors who specialize in sports medicine?

A: Yes, some orthopaedic surgeons, physiatrists, and other physicians choose to specialize in athletic injuries. The most well-known of these are team physicians to professional football, baseball, basketball, and hockey teams. However, although the experience of these specialists may ultimately be greater, their initial training is the same as any qualified specialist, and the techniques they use are similar to those employed in the general practice of orthopaedics. Any qualified orthopaedic surgeon or other such specialist is capable of diagnosing and treating the average sports injury. Further information on the practice of orthopaedics as well as a selection of informational brochures can be obtained from the American Academy of Orthopaedic Surgeons, 6300 N. River Road, Rosemont, IL 60018, phone (847) 823-7186.

Q: Why is the use of steroids by athletes banned?

A: The Canadian runner Ben Johnson had to give back the gold medal he won in the 24th Olympic Games for using steroids. This sent a clear message to the world that the use of steroids has no place in athletic competitions.

These drugs reduce body fat and increase muscle tissue. They help decrease the recovery time of muscles between workouts, thus allowing for more strenuous work-outs and giving an unfair competitive advantage. They also have a chemical effect on the brain that produces a sense of well-being, which is frequently associated with increased aggression. Continued use can cross the line into addiction.

Steroids are dangerous because they can lead to premature weakening of the arteries, stroke or heart attack, baldness, sterility, liver cancer, acne, personality changes, and cessation of menstruation, to mention but a few of their more serious side effects. Finally, the same muscle-building results may be obtained from using electrical stimulation. This technique, thought to be used by the Soviets for some time, is safer than drugs or hormones and is not illegal.

Q: Do you decondition as fast as you condition?

A: No, you decondition faster than you condition. At least twice as fast, sometimes even more rapidly, and especially if you are ill. The longer you are away from a conditioning program, the harder it is to get back in shape.

Q: Why is an injured joint stiff in the morning?

A: With inactivity, the tissues around the joint swell, causing stiffness. This swelling is relieved with movement during the day as motion squeezes the fluid away from the involved joint.

Q: My hip snaps and feels like it is loose. What causes this?

A: It is probably a tendon (usually the iliotibial band tendon) snapping over the greater trochanter (the bony protuberance at the side of the hip). When this happens, it feels as though your hip is actually slipping out of place. No need to worry, it isn't. Strengthening the muscle or stretching the tendon can sometimes be helpful. Occasionally a corrective operation is necessary.

Q: How do I know if I have a rotator cuff tear?

A: Rotator cuff tears occur in people who do a lot of activities that involve overhead use of the arms, such as tennis, swimming, and sports that involve throwing. Minimal tears usually do not cause any trouble in the amateur athlete. Larger tears can cause persistent pain, weakness, and even an inability to raise the arm to the forward elevated or side elevated position. You can all but ignore your rotator cuff tear if your shoulder does not hurt and you don't have a serious compromise in function, and if you keep your shoulder strong with appropriate exercises.

Q: My doctor wants to perform an operation to correct an athletic injury to my elbow. What are some of the questions I should be asking him before consenting to surgery?

A: Always inquire about nonsurgical alternatives. If such exist, ask why they aren't tried before surgery. You should also ask what the odds are that the operation will work, and if it can make you worse. Before consenting to surgery you should know what postsurgical rehabilitation is necessary. Finally, it is usually a good idea to get a second opinion regarding anticipated surgery.

Q: In general, what symptoms should alert an athlete to the possibility of an injury?

A: Any joint pain, tenderness, reduced motion, weakness, swelling, numbness, or tingling in an extremity would indicate the possibility of an injury that should not be ignored.

Q: What is reflex sympathetic dystrophy (RSD)?

A: RSD is a condition of decreased circulation to a part of the limb due to spasm of the blood vessels. It can cause serious damage, resulting in bone loss, limb atrophy and contracture, and unremitting pain. It can occur even after a minor injury. Its exact cause is unknown. To be successful, treatment must be started immediately and includes vigorous exercise of the involved part as well as intensive physical therapy, sympathetic nerve blocks, and certain medications.

7

Posture

Posture follows motion like a shadow. All movement begins and ends in posture.

Sir Charles Sherrington (1857–1952)

Many chronic orthopaedic complaints are aggravated or even caused by poor posture. Backache, neckache, tension, and fatigue may be related to poor standing, sitting, or lying postural habits. Orthopaedic problems of the spine (such as scoliosis) or pelvis (such as pelvic tilt), arthritis, and osteoporosis all can be aggravated by poor posture. Proper standing posture can reduce pressure on your joints, increase your available energy, make you more comfortable, and improve your attitude and self-confidence. Postural exercises can increase strength, endurance, and flexibility in your spine and limbs. Following a few simple rules of body mechanics will allow you to move, lift, and bend in the safest, most effective, and efficient way throughout your active working day.

The upright body is always fighting the force of gravity. The gravest (sic!) postural problems would all but disappear on the moon. Proper standing posture centers the weight of your torso over your pelvis and minimizes the problems caused by gravity. A plumb line (the line of gravity) dropped from your head falls behind your hips and through or just in front of your knees (Figure 7-1). The pelvis is slightly rotated forward, thus unloading and relaxing your hips and back. The abdomen is tight and flat, providing support in front for the lumbar spine. The position is relaxed and feels good. With the

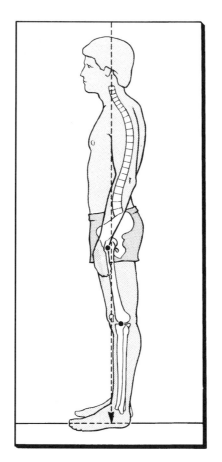

FIGURE 7-1   The Plumb Line of Gravity

plumb line falling behind the hips and in front of the knees, no stabilizing muscular action is necessary at these joints to maintain the upright posture. This is the most efficient stance, as it can be maintained with the expenditure of very little body energy. It is also the position from which actions such as stepping or jumping can be quickly initiated. Learn to be aware of your body and to develop a feeling of when it is in balance.

Figure 7-2 is a 60-second isometric work-out that will strengthen and tone your muscles and can be done while seated. Hold your breath while doing each exercise, and do each one for six seconds. Relax completely for a few seconds, and then go on to the next.

1. Pull-up (for arms and shoulders). Sitting straight, grasp the chair sides tightly with both hands and pull up as hard as possible.

2. Hand press (for arms, chest, and shoulders). Sitting straight with chest out and arms held across chest, place one fist inside the other. Press together using all the strength of your arms and shoulders.

3. Back pull (for the back). Keeping the back straight, lean forward until you can grasp your legs or braces of the chair, then pull straight up using only your back muscles.

4. Neck presser (for the neck). Sit straight, clasp your hands behind your neck holding your elbows forward. Pull forward with your hands and at the same time press your head backwards.

FIGURE 7-2a

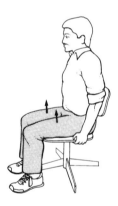

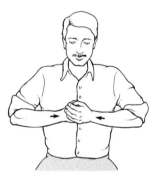

1

2

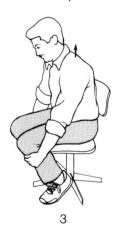

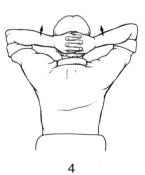

3

4

5. Stomach tightener (for waist and abdomen). Sit with your legs together straight out. Bend forward and grasp your legs just below the knees. Press down with the hands and at the same time press up against the hands with both legs.

6. Criss-cross (for chest and legs). Set the feet about four inches apart and bend forward, placing your hands against the inside of opposite knees. While attempting to press the knees together at the same time, hold them apart with the hands.

7. Body lift (for shoulders, arms, and abdomen). Keep your back straight. Now lean forward and place your hands, palms down, against the side of the chair. Holding your legs straight out, attempt to raise your body about one inch off the chair.

8. Leg squeezer (for thighs and calves). Sit forward on the edge of the chair. Leaning back, hold your legs straight out. Hook one foot over the other and hold them tightly together. Resting your feet on the floor, keep your legs straight and try to pull the

FIGURE 7-2b

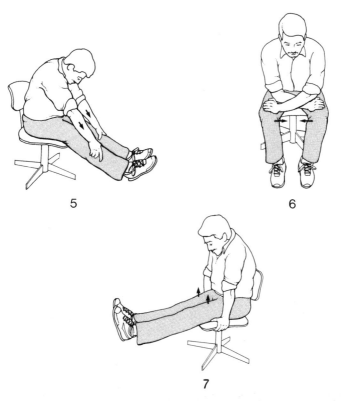

5

6

7

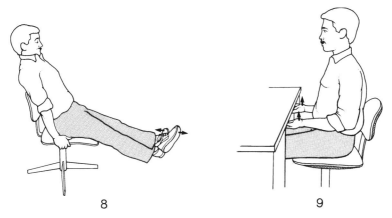

FIGURE 7-2c

your feet on the floor, keep your legs straight and try to pull the feet apart.

9. Arm curl (for the upper arms). Sitting straight, grasp the underside of a heavy table or desk with your palms up and your forearms parallel to the desk. Push up as hard as possible.

Following is a list of rules for maintaining good posture during motion, thus avoiding injury through proper balance and efficient movement.

1. Always lift from the knees (Figure 7-3), keeping the back straight. Keep the load close to you, and use your abdominal muscles, not those of your back. Lift with your legs.

FIGURE 7-3 Proper Lifting Technique

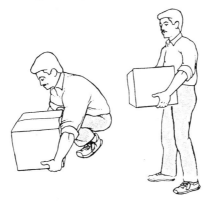

1. Always lift from the knees
2. Hold the load close to your body

2. When reaching, keep the back straight and support yourself firmly on your legs. Bend the knees.

3. When bending over, keep your head and neck in line with your back. Bend from the knees and keep the abdomen tight to support the lumbar spine.

4. If possible, do all work at eye or waist level, never when looking up. When standing for prolonged periods (such as at an ironing board or sink), elevate one foot on a small stool or thick phone book. This will flatten the low back and relieve strain.

5. Sit in straight, firm chairs, using a lumbar support to bolster the low back (Figure 7-4). This can be a small firm pillow or a rolled up towel placed in the small of the back. Chair height can be adjusted to shift the weight forward off the spine and keep the arms at desk level. The feet should be kept flat on the floor, with the buttocks flush against the back of the chair. Position ought to be shifted frequently during the day.

6. Turning should be done with the whole body rather than just at the waist, especially when shifting weight from one surface to another.

7. When walking, try to make the very top of your head touch the sky or ceiling. The shoulders should be thrown back and the abdomen pulled tight.

8. Although position is difficult to control while sleeping, using pillows under the knees can relax the hip and back muscles. Of course, the mattress must be firm (Figure 7-5).

FIGURE 7-4   Good Sitting Posture—Keep your shoulders back, stomach in, head up, and feet flat on the floor

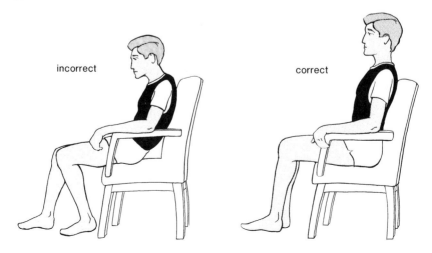

incorrect   correct

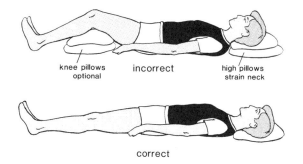

knee pillows   incorrect   high pillows
 optional   strain neck

correct

FIGURE 7-5   Good Lying Posture—Lie flat on your back—use only a small pillow

POSTURAL EXERCISES

1. *For the neck*: Six position isometric neck exercises (see chapter on the neck) are useful for maintaining strength in the neck. Neck rotations and stretching forward, backward, and to either side will maintain neck flexibility.

2. *For the shoulders*: Touching the shoulder tips to the ears and trying to touch the shoulder blades by throwing the shoulders back can maintain flexibility in the shoulders. These exercises should be repeated at least a dozen times twice a day.

3. *For the low back*: Partial sit-ups with the knees bent are excellent for developing abdominal tone. Williams' exercises, detailed in the chapter on back care, can maintain suppleness in the low back.

GENERAL POSTURAL EXERCISES FOR THE NECK

1. *Neck glide*—Glide your head straight back, keeping your nose level with your ears. Hold for 15 counts and repeat 12 times.

2. *Neck stretch*—Tilt your head to one side, putting your left ear over its shoulder. Relax and let gravity pull your head down to stretch your neck. Hold for 12 counts and repeat on the opposite side.

FOR THE THORACIC (UPPER) SPINE

1. *Corner press*—Stand in a corner with a hand on each wall, at shoulder height. Press your chest against wall. Hold for a count of 15 and press back up. Repeat 12 times.

2. *Thoracic stretch*—Bend your elbows 90° at your side. Bring one arm above the other behind your neck as far as you can. Hold for a count of 15. Then bring that arm down and the other one overhead. Repeat 12 times.

FOR THE LUMBAR (LOW) SPINE

1. *Press up*—Lie face down with your hands shoulder width apart. Gently press up, bringing your head and chest up but keeping your hips on the floor. Hold for a count of 15, lower yourself, and repeat 12 times.

2. *Shoulder curl*—Lying on your back with your knees bent, keep your arms folded across your chest or abdomen. Lift your head, neck, and shoulders from the supporting surface. Hold for a count of 15 and repeat 12 times.

These exercises stretch and strengthen your cervical, thoracic, and lumbar spine.

Needless to say, many things other than slouching contribute to poor posture. Overweight (particularly a potbelly) is a major factor that adversely affects good posture. Walking with unbalanced loads and wearing improper shoes (particularly high heels, which strain the low back) also can lead to poor posture. Good posture can make you look, feel, and function better.

Poor posture is usually a *functional deformity,* that is to say, it can be corrected at will. However, not all postural deformities are functional. Some are structural (rigid) and require more than a change in habit or habitus for correction. One such is scoliosis, or curvature of the spine, which the next chapter will discuss.

QUESTIONS AND ANSWERS ABOUT POSTURE

Q: What is the study of "body mechanics?"
A: Body mechanics is the science of posture in motion. It teaches us the most efficient and safest ways to move, bend, reach, lift, stand, walk, and otherwise use our musculoskeletal system in all the motor activities we perform.
Q: What are the natural curves of the spine?
A: There are three (Figure 7-6): (1) the cervical spine has a lordotic (forward bowed) curve; (2) the thoracic spine has a kyphotic (bowed backward) curve; and (3) the lumbar spine has a lordotic curve. Exaggeration or reversal of these curves can inhibit good posture and cause pain.

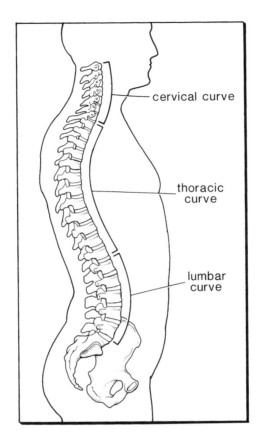

FIGURE 7-6   The Three Natural Curves of the Spine

Q: Why is the chapter on posture just about in the middle of this book?

A: Because healthy posture is central to all other considerations about bone. It guards against vertebral fracture and osteoporosis. It aligns and protects the body from arthritis. It provides the safest way to move to avoid falls, fractures, and soft tissue injuries. It enhances performance during sports activity. It safeguards against scoliosis. It decreases the incidence of low back and neck pain. It keeps the knees and feet aligned. It provides a solid base for use of the hands.

Q: What can computer operators, secretaries, and other workers who sit all day do to avoid postural strain?

A: Following the general rules outlined in this chapter will help. The use of a lumbar support (a lumbar roll or a towel rolled up to 4 to 6 inches in diameter) placed against the small of the back can relieve strain in the lumbar curve. Chair height can be adjusted so that weight is shifted forward off the spine. Adjust the seat angle to avoid undue pressure on your legs just above the knees, and avoid crossing your legs while working, because this can constrict circulation. The computer monitor should be at the height of your forehead so you are looking straight ahead. You should view the monitor from a distance of from 18 to 24 inches. The arms should be at desk level, with a table height of between 2 and 2.5 feet, adjusted so that when using your keyboard your elbows will be bent 90 degrees and your wrists will lie flat. A wrist pad can make this position more comfortable. Use your entire arm to move a mouse device, and position your mouse pad within comfortable reach. A small wedge on the seat may be required. Position ought to be shifted during the day to keep the muscles loose and to relax away any tension built up due to immobility. The feet should be kept flat on the floor to maintain good sitting posture. This also aids leg circulation. A foot rest may be necessary. Finally, remember to relax and take frequent short breaks from your work—lean back and breathe deeply, stand, and stretch. Both your body and mind will benefit from such a routine.

8

Scoliosis

As the twig is bent so grows the tree, as the spine is bent so grows the child.

Anon.

The term *scoliosis* refers to an abnormal curvature of the spine. The most common types occur in late childhood, although scoliosis can be present at birth and adult forms are seen.

The spine has two normal mild curves when viewed from the side, one in the upper thoracic area that rounds out the shoulder region, the other in the low back or lumbar area—the normal lumbar lordosis (Greek: I bend). The normal spine is perfectly straight when viewed from the front or back. Scoliosis produces a curve (or curves) to the right and/or left so that the spine is not straight when viewed from in front or behind (Figure 8-1).

In order to compensate for such a curve, the pelvis will tilt and the hips and shoulders may become uneven. The spine may also rotate, giving one-sided prominence to the ribs and leading to a rib hump on one side of the back. Such deformity may initially be passively correctable, but eventually there will be bony structural change that leads to wedging and other permanent malformation of the vertebral bodies.

People with scoliosis may also show an increased rounding of their shoulders, or a sway-back. Again, these deformations may initially be passively correctable but later become fixed. Although there are many notable scoliotics in history and literature (consider, for example, Steinmetz, the renowned scientific electrical genius, and Richard III, King of England, known as

103

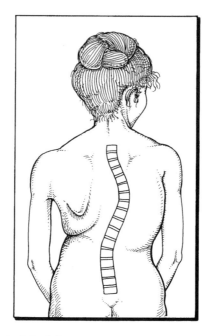

FIGURE 8-1 Scoliotic Spinal Curve

"crouchback," the subject of a tragedy by Shakespeare), the most famous may well be Quasimodo, the Hunchback of Notre Dame in Victor Hugo's novel, *Notre Dame de Paris.*

There are many causes of scoliosis. They include:

❏ *Postural,* (or *functional) scoliosis* is due to poor standing and sitting habitus. These curves are minimal and correct themselves when the child is lying down.

❏ *Transient scoliosis* may be due to irritation of nerve roots from slipped disc or any other inflammation. It resolves with correction of the inciting condition.

❏ *Structural scoliosis.* There are several types, including:

1. Idiopathic scoliosis comprises more than 70 percent of all cases. It may be genetic and can occur from infancy to adolescence. Girls are affected more often than boys. The cause of this type of scoliosis is unknown.
2. Congenital scoliosis is probably not genetic. It is often associated with other spinal defects.
3. Scoliosis may be caused by neuromuscular diseases such as muscular dystrophy, cerebral palsy, or poliomyelitis.

4. Scoliosis may occur as the result of injury, such as fractures of the vertebrae or injuries to the thorax.
5. Scoliosis may be due to other diseases, such as various types of dwarfism, rheumatoid arthritis, osteogenesis imperfecta, or neurofibromatosis.

EVALUATION OF THE PATIENT WITH SCOLIOSIS

A complete history is taken, paying special attention to any contributory causes, such as other disorders or diseases that may be related to the scoliosis. The age of discovery of the abnormal spinal curve is noted, which may be considerably later than the age of onset. Scoliosis does not cause pain in children, and its first indication may be difficulty in fitting clothes.

Many cases of scoliosis are initially picked up in school screening programs, which should be a routine part of the physical examination of schoolchildren. This is a considerable challenge as there are over 20 million children between the ages of 9 and 15 in the United States. Scoliosis screening programs are important because, as a rule, the earlier scoliosis is detected the more successful is the treatment.

Another important part of the history is determining the state of secondary sexual development in the patient. Idiopathic curves commonly stop progressing at the time spinal growth is complete. This typically occurs by age 15 in girls and 16 in boys.

Physical examination evaluates and measures not only the curve, including its rotation, but also the state of the heart and lungs, which can be compromised by an advanced spinal curvature. Progression of scoliosis can be very rapid, particularly during growth spurts such as that seen in the early teens.

X-rays of the spine, usually taken standing, enable the physician to measure the curve and follow its progress. That spinal growth is complete can be ascertained by the status of growth plates in the vertebrae, pelvis, and ribs, and by an estimation of bony age by x-raying the bones of the wrist and comparing them to a standard atlas of bone growth. This is necessary because bone age may not necessarily coincide with chronologic age.

Pulmonary function can be evaluated by measuring lung volume as well as oxygenation of the blood.

TREATMENT

The best treatment for scoliosis is early detection. Most spinal curves can be treated without surgery if they are detected before they become severe. A simple examination of the child stripped to the waist and bending forward will reveal any asymmetry of the back, and suspect cases can be referred for further examination and x-ray. Any time a spinal deformity is detected in a child, all of his or her siblings should be examined because of the possibility of heredity playing a role in causation.

Although an exercise program may improve muscular tone about the spine, it cannot correct scoliosis and should always be augmented by bracing or surgery.

Braces can be used to control mild curves in growing children. These braces *(spinal orthoses)* have been improved to the point where state-of-the-art appliances are now low profile and can be worn underneath ordinary clothing. A brace will not usually correct a curved spine, rather it is used solely to keep the scoliosis from rapidly progressing. Some braces, such as the Milwaukee brace, are designed to be used with specific exercises while wearing the appliance.

SCOLIOSIS EXERCISES

1. *Pelvic tilt*—Lie on your back with both knees bent up and the feet placed flat. Tighten your stomach muscles and roll your hips back so as to flatten the small of the back into the bed. Hold for count of 5. Relax and repeat.

2. *Knee to chest*—Lie on your back with both knees bent up, then raise one knee at a time to chest, alternating knees.

3. *Partial sit-up*—Lie on your back with both knees bent up, reach your hands toward the knees and raise your head and shoulders.

4. *Lower trunk rotation*—Lying on your back with both knees bent up, roll your knees from side to side.

5. *Lateral leg lift*—Lying on your (left/right) side, slightly bend the bottom leg, raising the top leg up straight. You can also do this exercise with a small towel roll under your rib cage.

6. *Upper trunk side bending*—Bend to the left/right side while sitting or standing with hands on your hips.

7. *Upper trunk rotation*—Sitting or standing with hands on your hips, rotate toward the (left/right) side pulling (left/right) shoulder back.

8. *Cat / Camel*—Get on your hands and knees, then alternate arching the back up as high as you can and sinking down as low as you can.

9. *Unilateral extension*—On your hands and knees, raise the opposite arm and leg (right arm/left leg; left arm/right leg), alternating side to side.

10. *Prone extension*—Lying on your stomach, raise one arm at a time, then both arms, one leg at a time, then both legs.

11. *Prone push-ups*—Lying on your stomach with hands beside your head, push up, keeping your hips on the supporting surface and bending at small of back.

12. *Handwalking*—On your hands and knees, sit back on your heels and walk your hands to (left/right) side.

Most braces are worn for 23 hours a day and removed only for bathing or swimming. Swimming is an excellent exercise for the scoliotic patient, as it utilizes spinal motion in an essentially weightless situation. Plaster casts have also been employed in the treatment of scoliosis. This involves positioning the patient on a special plaster table where traction and pressure on the spine correct the curve before the plaster is applied.

Electrical stimulation of the muscles of the back has been used to treat some mild scoliotic curves. Stimulation is applied only at night and avoids the inconvenience of wearing a brace while sleeping. This treatment is not applicable to all spinal curves.

SURGERY

Some curves progress to the point where they can only be treated surgically. An attempt to achieve maximum correction with traction before surgery is sometimes made. Surgery is indicated when the deformity is severe enough to threaten pulmonary or cardiac function, when it can no longer be controlled with conservative treatment, when it is considerable enough to present an unwanted cosmetic appearance, or when it is painful.

Surgery consists of spinal fusion with bone grafts, usually taken from the back of the patient's pelvis or specially processed bone and/or bone substitute. Spinal fusion can be accomplished from the front or the back of the spine, sometimes both. A variety of mechanical devices may be used to augment the fusion and hold the spine in a corrected position until the graft heals and the fusion is solid. These devices distract or compress the vertebrae or wire them to long supporting metal rods, maintaining rigid fixation and support of the corrected curve. With modern surgical and recovery room techniques, patients easily survive these operations; they are sitting upright within days and are released from the hospital after a brief postoperative stay. Because of the mechanical fixation devices used, braces or casts are seldom required after surgery.

Scoliosis in adults can occur secondary to osteoarthritis. Surgery is sometimes necessary to relieve pain and lessen disability.

Although the cause of much scoliosis is still unknown, early recognition and prompt treatment utilizing state-of-the-art techniques can in most instances prevent progression of the curve, granting the child with scoliosis the promise of normal appearance and function. For the time being, let's stick with the back but consider a problem less serious but much more common than scoliosis. What I will talk about next is low back pain.

QUESTIONS AND ANSWERS ABOUT SCOLIOSIS

Q: Can exercises alone correct scoliosis?

A: No, but properly supervised exercise can keep the spine supple so that it is more easily corrected by bracing or surgery.

Q: Why is congenital scoliosis (scoliosis at birth) often severe and difficult to correct?

A: Because congenital scoliosis almost always involves anomalies of the vertebrae. That is, partial or poor development of the bony elements of the spine.

Q: At what age does *idiopathic* scoliosis usually become apparent?

A: Most cases of idiopathic scoliosis become apparent in late puberty or early adolescence as a result of the rapid growth spurt that the body (and spine) undergoes at this time.

Q: How does one determine when bony growth is complete?

A: By x-raying bony *physes* (growth plates) to see when they fuse to the rest of the bone. The epiphyseal growth plate at the wrist is most commonly observed. Manuals illustrating the status of the physes at the wrist at monthly intervals until skeletal growth has been complete are available for this purpose. In the case of scoliosis, one also looks at the growth plates of the ribs and vertebrae as well as a special growth plate that caps the pelvic brim.

9

Low Back Pain

The belly robs the back!

Dutch Proverb

The National Insurance Council reports that low back injury is second only to the common cold as a cause of work loss in the United States. More than 100 million workdays are lost each year, and billions of dollars are paid out in lawsuit awards, disability claims, and other settlements resulting from back disability. The American Academy of Orthopaedic Surgeons calculates that more than three billion dollars is spent annually in the U.S. on the diagnosis and treatment of lumbar disc disorders. Several billion dollars more go to the physical therapists, chiropractors, acupuncturists, and a variety of other "therapists" who promote more exotic cures. The total bill for lost work time, tests, treatment, legal fees and awards, medications, and back products is therefore in excess of eighty billion dollars a year!

This means that most people will at some time experience a backache. It is so frequent that economic losses because of absenteeism due to low back pain exceed 24 billion dollars every year. Why is this so? The answer is that, although we are designed for standing and walking, we perform both activities with an incredible mix of strengths *and* weaknesses.

We are born with a relatively straight spine, then develop a curve in the low back at about one year of age. This builds some "spring" into the spinal column to compensate for the jarring that occurs with ordinary walking. The fact that the spine is made of many small stacked bones instead of one massive bony column allows for all the turning and bending to which it is subject. Romans called this spine the vertebral column—"vertebral" means "turning" in Latin. The word *vertigo* comes from the same root.

Standing frees the arms for functional tasks and allows the now-upright creature to see farther than he could when crouched on all fours. These are both positive evolutionary survival features. As an aside, the springy backbone each of us has is stretched out in the morning because of the horizontal sleeping posture, which makes us taller at 7 o'clock in the morning than we are at the same time in the evening.

However, there are disadvantages to standing. When misapplied, the long lever arm of the back can exert forces up to 1,500 pounds per square inch on any of the vertebral bodies or, worse yet, the cushioning discs that lie between them (Figure 9-1). Sedentary posture causes stress because the highest measured pressure inside the disc occurs with sitting; it is even higher than when standing or walking. That is why the highest risk groups for back pain are people who spend a lot of time sitting and leaning forward—clerks, truck drivers, and the like.

Also contributing to spinal instability is the protruding midriff ("the belly robs the back!") that seems to be an almost inevitable accompaniment of middle age. Standing is not optimal in terms of the pull on our internal organs. Four-footed animals have their organs "slung from a pole," whereas ours are hung from a pole. Without reinforcement from the front, the tug of the abdominal organs on the back can exert considerable chronic stress on both the bones and surrounding soft tissues (ligaments, tendons, and muscles). Poor posture provokes the mechanical problems that initiate and perpetuate low back pain, particularly when aggravated by obesity and lack of regular exercise.

Most low back pain is caused by injury sustained from improper posture, poor sleeping or sitting habits, or incorrect bending or lifting techniques. Some back problems are the result of sports injuries or motor accidents. Infection or tumors can also cause back pain; these problems must be ruled out during the orthopaedic examination. Low back pain can also be

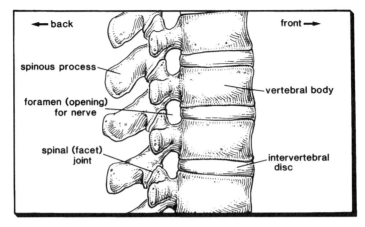

FIGURE 9-1   Normal Vertebrae

caused by fractures to vertebrae, particularly in the osteoporotic spine and commonly found in the lower part of the back, as well as by arthritic conditions. Scoliosis usually does not cause pain, but arthritis secondary to spinal curvature can be uncomfortable. Another back condition, called "spondylolisthesis" (*spondylo:* back; *listhesis:* slipping) is a cleft in the structure of the rear part of a vertebral body that creates instability, causing one vertebra to slip on another. This may be due to a congenital anomaly, a stress fracture, or even an acute break. Spondylolisthesis is found in approximately 2 percent of the population and is amenable to surgical stabilization.

Finally, emotional stress can cause or aggravate low back pain. It is not by chance that the common slang we use includes such admonitions as "get off my back!" or "this job is breaking my back!" Camptocormia (from the Greek *kamptein,* to bend; *kournes,* the trunk) is a form of hysteria, seen most often in soldiers. It is characterized by extreme bending of the back, the eyes usually being focused on the ground. The expression of emotional tension through physical symptoms is called *somatization,* and people indeed tend to displace their tensions to their spinal column, resulting in pain in both the neck and the low back.

Pain in the low back commonly results from damage to the soft tissues, such as overstretched ligaments or crushed discs. The intervertebral disc is a soft cushion between the vertebrae. Under strain, a disc may bulge and press on one or several of the nerves to the leg (Figure 9-2). The most severe form of such

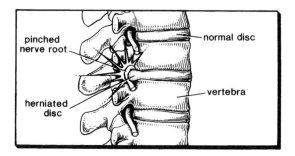

FIGURE 9-2   Herniated Disc

injury is a herniated or ruptured disc. In this condition, the restraining margin of the disc is torn and the thick, jelly-like disc material pushes out, pressing on a spinal nerve. Pain from this type of injury travels from the back to the foot; this is called sciatica.

The more common "lumbago" is back strain. This was called a hexen-shuss or kick from a witch in times gone by, and was often treated with various primitive methods designed to get rid of the witch.

History and physical examination are the mainstay of the diagnosis of low back pain. As noted, the history is usually one of an effort strain to the low back. Pain and muscle spasm are commonly experienced, and may be referred down one or both legs. Pain and numbness experienced as far as the toes can indicate a protruding or herniated intervertebral disc. However, pain from muscle spasm alone can be referred down the back of the legs as far as the knees.

Examination will reveal limitation of motion in the back and often a painful shift of the torso over the pelvis. Changing position may be difficult and straight leg raising from the supine position will elicit pain in the back or down the leg. In the case of pressure on the sciatic nerve from a protruding disc or other pathology, the deep tendon reflex at the knee or ankle can be depressed or absent and a typical distribution of loss of sensation will be seen.

Laboratory tests may include an x-ray of the lumbosacral spine. Bony abnormalities may be noted on these x-rays. Narrowing of the disc space should be present if the disc is protruding or herniated. Other testing may be ordered in individual cases, including examination of the blood for evidence of arthritis, infection, or other contributing causes. Electrical examination of nerve and muscle function (electromyography and nerve conduction velocity) can provide information about nerve damage. A *computed tomographic (CT) scan* can reveal pathology such as tumor or disc protrusion, and *myelography* (an x-ray of the spine after the introduction of a radiopaque contrast material into the spinal fluid) should further localize a herniated disc or other space-occupying pathology. A bone scan involves visualizing uptake by the bones of a radiopaque material that has been injected into the bloodstream; it can localize pathology, particularly infection, fracture, arthritis, or tumor. *Magnetic resonance imaging (MRI)* is a state-of-the-art-technique that visualizes bone but particularly soft tissues of the spine and is very useful in the diagnosis of pathology of these structures, particularly the intervertebral discs.

TREATMENT OF LOW BACK PAIN

The most important part of the treatment of low back pain is proper posture. This does not mean military posture or standing straight all the time. It refers to a relaxed and balanced stance and gait so that the torso is well seated over the pelvis. The important thing is to avoid a curve or sway-back in the lumbar spine. To do this, you must elevate one leg on a small stool (a thick phone book will do) whenever standing for any period of time. Never—repeat, never—bend from the waist; always bend from the knees and hips. When lifting a heavy object, hold it close to you. Remember that the weight of the torso alone can exert a force of more than 1,500 pounds per square inch on the intervertebral discs of the low back when you bend improperly. You should never bend over without bending the knees.

Homemakers are at particular risk when performing household chores. They should change from one task to another before their back becomes strained. Body position should be checked frequently. What you are looking for is a flat back and a tight abdomen. You can sense this position by standing away from a wall, then leaning with your back against the wall, bending the knees slightly and tightening the abdomen, thus tilting your pelvis and flatting the lower spine while you shimmy up the wall to the standing position.

Horses don't have to worry about back pain. Not only do they get around on all fours, but through a unique system of interlocking ligaments and bones in their legs, which serve as a sling to suspend their body weight without strain while their muscles are completely relaxed, they can stand continuously for as long as a month. Because horses are heavy but have relatively fragile bones, lying in one position for a long time can cause muscle cramping.

Chairs should be designed to prevent slumping and provide support for the low back. Having the knees higher than the hips relaxes the back. Strain may be relieved by sitting forward, again flattening the back by tightening the abdominal muscles and crossing the knees. Slumping in a chair leads to strain not only of the low back but also of the neck and shoulders. The chair you use should provide firm comfortable seating.

You should sleep on an extra-firm mattress. If you have any doubt as to the firmness of the sleeping surface, a bedboard (3/4 inch plywood cut to size or a commercial bedboard) can be slipped between the mattress and the bedspring. Contrary to mattress advertising, the purpose of a firm mattress is not so much to support you during sleep as to prevent you from sleeping in one position for too long. The soft tissues of the back are viscoelastic and tend to "gel" when they are not stretched. This leads to stiffness and "morning backache." A small pillow should be used; a high one places strain on the neck and shoulders. Although sleeping habits are difficult to change, sleeping on the side or the back is more conducive to back support and good posture than is sleeping on the stomach. Raising the foot of the mattress slightly can discourage the abdominal sleeping position.

When the back is tired or painful, lying down on a firm carpeted floor with two bolsters or cushions from a couch or lounge chair to elevate the knees will relieve spinal strain. Mild exercises (Williams' exercises) that will stretch and strengthen the back are illustrated in Figure 9-3. Isometric exercises are also useful. Here is a good one: As frequently as you can during the day, usually while waiting for a traffic light, bus, and so forth, tighten your abdomen while trying to touch your navel to your backbone. Hold this for a count of six, then relax. Practice breathing normally with the abdomen tight. This can be done while sitting or standing. This exercise is not only useful for the back but in several weeks you also should take an inch off your waistline.

Remember not to strain your back. *Always* bend from the hips and knees, never from the waist. Avoid carrying unbalanced loads, and never carry anything heavier than you can easily manage. Avoid sudden movements. Try to keep your head in line with your spine. Wear shoes that have moderate heels.

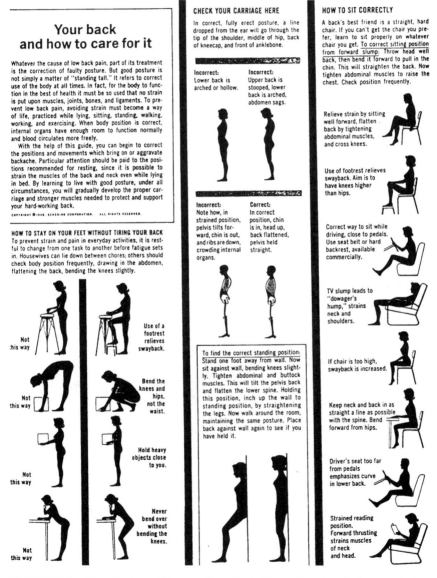

FIGURE 9-3 Your Back and How to Care for It (Reproduced with the permission of Schering Corporation, Copyright © 1965. All rights reserved.)

HOW TO PUT YOUR BACK TO BED

For proper bed posture, a firm mattress is essential. Bedboards, sold commercially, or devised at home, may be used with soft mattresses. Bedboards, preferably, should be made of ¾ inch plywood. Faulty sleeping positions intensify swayback and result not only in backache but in numbness, tingling, and pain in arms and legs.

Incorrect:
Lying flat on back makes swayback worse.

Correct:
Lying on side with knees bent effectively flattens the back. Flat pillow may be used to support neck, especially when shoulders are broad.

Use of high pillow strains neck, arms, shoulders.

Sleeping on back is restful and correct when knees are properly supported.

Sleeping face down exaggerates swayback, strains neck and shoulders.

Raise the foot of the mattress eight inches to discourage sleeping on the abdomen.

Bending one hip and knee does not relieve swayback.

Proper arrangement of pillows for resting or reading in bed.

A straight-back chair used behind a pillow makes a serviceable backrest.

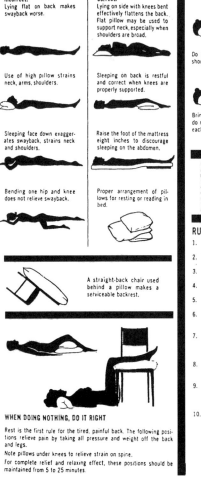

WHEN DOING NOTHING, DO IT RIGHT

Rest is the first rule for the tired, painful back. The following positions relieve pain by taking all pressure and weight off the back and legs.

Note pillows under knees to relieve strain on spine.

For complete relief and relaxing effect, these positions should be maintained from 5 to 25 minutes.

EXERCISE—WITHOUT GETTING OUT OF BED
Exercises to be performed while lying in bed are aimed not so much at strengthening muscles as at teaching correct positioning. But muscles used correctly become stronger and in time are able to support the body with the least amount of effort.

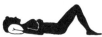

Do all exercises in this position. Legs should not be straightened.

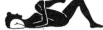

Bring knee up to chest. Lower slowly but do not straighten leg. Relax. Repeat with each leg 10 times.

Bring both knees slowly up to chest. Tighten muscles of abdomen, press back flat against bed. Hold knees to chest 20 seconds, then lower slowly. Relax. Repeat 5 times. This exercise gently stretches the shortened muscles of the lower back, while strengthening abdominal muscles. Clasp knees, bring them up to chest, at the same time coming to a sitting position. Rock back and forth.

EXERCISE—WITHOUT ATTRACTING ATTENTION
Use these inconspicuous exercises whenever you have a spare moment during the day, both to relax tension and improve the tone of important muscle groups.

1. Rotate shoulders, forward and backward.
2. Turn head slowly side to side.
3. Watch an imaginary plane take off, just below the right shoulder. Stretch neck, follow it slowly as it moves up, around and down, disappearing below the other shoulder. Repeat, starting on left side.
4. Slowly, slowly, touch left ear to left shoulder; right ear to right shoulder. Raise both shoulders to touch ears, drop them as far down as possible.
5. At any pause in the day — waiting for an elevator to arrive, for a specific traffic light to change — pull in abdominal muscles, tighten, hold it for the count of eight without breathing. Relax slowly. Increase the count gradually after the first week, practice breathing normally with the abdomen flat and contracted. Do this sitting, standing, and walking.

RULES TO LIVE BY—FROM NOW ON

1. Never bend from the waist only; bend the hips and knees.
2. Never lift a heavy object higher than your waist.
3. Always turn and face the object you wish to lift.
4. Avoid carrying unbalanced loads; hold heavy objects close to your body.
5. Never carry anything heavier than you can manage with ease.
6. Never lift or move heavy furniture. Wait for someone to do it who knows the principles of leverage.
7. Avoid sudden movements, sudden "overloading" of muscles. Learn to move deliberately, swinging the legs from the hips.
8. Learn to keep the head in line with the spine, when standing, sitting, lying in bed.
9. Put soft chairs and deep couches on your "don't sit" list. During prolonged sitting, cross your legs to rest your back.
10. Your doctor is the only one who can determine when low back pain is due to faulty posture. He is the best judge of when you may do general exercises for physical fitness. When you do, omit any exercise which arches or overstrains the lower back, backward bends, or forward bends, touching the toes with the knees straight.
11. Wear shoes with moderate heels, all about the same height. Avoid changing from high to low heels.
12. Put a footrail under the desk, and a footrest under the crib.
13. Diaper the baby sitting next to him or her on the bed.
14. Don't stoop and stretch to hang the wash; raise the clothesbasket and lower the washline.
15. Beg or buy a rocking chair. Rocking rests the back by changing the muscle groups used.
16. Train yourself vigorously to use your abdominal muscles to flatten your lower abdomen. In time, this muscle contraction will become habitual, making you the envied possessor of a youthful body-profile!
17. Don't strain to open windows or doors.
18. For good posture, concentrate on strengthening "nature's corset"—the abdominal and buttock muscles. The pelvic roll exercise is especially recommended to correct the postural relation between the pelvis and the spine.

FIGURE 9-3   (Continued).

Do not stoop or stretch without thinking of your back. Remember that using a rocking chair rests the back by changing muscle groups used during various times of the rocking cycle. For good posture, concentrate on strengthening your abdomen and your buttocks. The pelvic tilt exercise is particularly recommended for proper back posture. The use of an appropriate support for the back while riding in a car (sometimes just a small wedge pillow will do) will go a long way toward preventing back strain.

Do not forget that your mind set has a great deal to do with pain. Try to clear your life of stressful situations that lead to muscular tension. Some exercises are better than others for back pain. Swimming is excellent because of the body's weightless state in water. Biking is good, as is walking (in proper shoes on cinder or springy turf). Jogging is out, as is any other athletic activity that involves twisting or cutting, thus causing sudden low back stress.

GIVE YOUR BACK A BREAK

1. Avoid bending from the low back. Bend only from the knees.

2. Do not lift heavy objects, particularly overhead. All work should be performed at eye or waist level.

3. Use a firm mattress. Insert a bedboard (3/4 inch thick plywood or commercial bedboard) between the mattress and the springs.

4. Use firm or semi-firm chairs that support the low back.

5. Apply some heat (hot shower, hot tub soak, heating pad [on low], hot water bottle, and so forth) to the low back for at least 15 minutes twice a day.

6. At rest, elevate your knees and legs with several bolsters from the sofa, thus flexing the hips and relaxing the back.

7. Use a small wedge pillow to support the back when riding in a car.

Here are some tips for obtaining relief when back pain does occur. Medication such as aspirin or some of the other nonprescription anti-inflammatory drugs can be used to control short-term pain flareups. Ice will reduce inflammation and help to break the pain cycle. Commercial ice packs or even a sack of frozen vegetables can be applied for 15 to 20 minutes two to three times a day. Heat may also relieve pain and relax muscle. Moist heat is much more penetrating than dry, so showers, baths, and hot water bottles are particularly recommended. If you have access to a whirlpool, this is better yet.

Rest is a very important part of the conservative care of backache. Spasm and pain are the body's way of telling you that you should rest. Physical therapy is sometimes prescribed by a doctor. This usually includes heat (infrared or short-wave diathermy), massage, ultrasound, and sometimes pelvic traction. A therapist may recommend electrical stimulation with a "TENS" unit, which is worn by the patient and activated to stimulate nerve to relieve pain.

Your physician is the only one who can make a diagnosis and initiate an appropriate program of therapy for a backache that does not rapidly respond to the simple measures outlined here. The recommended treatment will depend on the cause of the back pain. It may simply be due to a muscular and ligamentous strain, or it may be due to a slipped or ruptured disc, arthritis, tension or emotional problems, or to something more serious, such as an infection or tumor. Recommendations may include physical therapy or manual therapy (manipulation of the spine), local injection of steroid or a nerve block, a body corset or brace, or pain-relieving medication, muscle relaxants, and nonsteroidal anti-inflammatory drugs. A back care program that teaches proper body mechanics can be initiated. Weight loss is often an important part of such a regimen, as is a closely supervised program of graded reconditioning exercise. Psychological evaluation may indicate mental stress that requires psychological therapy or counseling. All this may be directed through a so-called "back school program" or pain clinic.

Only about 10 percent of people who experience back pain ever require more than conservative treatment. The most common indications for surgery are disc protrusions or herniations, spinal stenosis (a narrowing of the bony canal that contains the spinal cord and its nerves), arthritis, or instability of the spine leading to nerve irritation. People with these conditions are often given a trial in hospital of intensive physical therapy, bed rest with traction, oral medications (usually nonsteroidal anti-inflammatory drugs, but sometimes steroids). An epidural steroid injection is often prescribed, in which liquid steroid (a potent anti-inflammatory medication) is injected into the area of nerve irritation, sometimes in combination with morphine. This may have to be repeated once or twice. In some cases, the injection has "cooled down" an inflamed nerve, thus avoiding the need for surgery. *Prolotherapy* involves injecting a solution that stiffens the soft tissue of the ligaments around the offending spinal segment, and it has been claimed that this provides spinal support. Acupuncture is becoming increasingly popular in the treatment of low back pain, as are other alternative or complementary medical therapies.

Several forms of surgical treatment are available. Chemonucleolysis involves injecting an enzyme similar to the papaya extract that is used in meat tenderizer, which dissolves the softer portion of the disc and allows the remainder to shrink and retract, thus taking pressure off the nerve. This procedure carries some risk (particularly if you are one of the unlucky few who happen to be allergic to the enzyme) and also requires considerable skill. Therefore it has generally fallen out of favor.

Surgery for a ruptured disc involves removal of enough bone in the back to expose and excise the ruptured portion of the disc, called a *laminotomy* (opening of the spinal lamina). A *laminectomy* involves removing the entire lamina, and is usually performed when spinal stenosis is present to gain access to the nerve roots in order to decompress them. Alternative operative methods in selected cases include using a microscope to excise a disc through a tiny "keyhole incision" (microdiscectomy) or sucking it out through a tiny cannula (percutaneous automated discectomy). Disc surgery using a small endoscope is also being tried experimentally. A *wide laminectomy* freeing the spinal cord and nerves is performed when spinal stenosis is present. For those cases in which instability is the primary problem, one way to fuse the spine and gain stability is wide bone grafting, usually with bone from the pelvis.

An ounce of prevention is worth a pound of cure, and this is especially true in the prevention and treatment of low back pain. To summarize, you can keep your back fit by maintaining good posture and following a well-balanced program of exercise, as well as by avoiding strain. You should avoid excessive swayback at all times, and always lift with your legs, not with your back. Sleeping and sitting habits are important. Taking some basic precautions and making some changes *now* can help you prevent serious back pain problems later. Severe or persistent back pain should be reported to your doctor, especially if you experience pain or numbness down either leg. Take charge of your back and you will stay out of trouble.

Now, how about that "pain in the neck?"

QUESTIONS AND ANSWERS ABOUT THE BACK

Q: If "the belly robs the back." what is the best exercise for strengthening the abdominal muscles?

A: Sit-ups or curl-ups are the best exercises for strengthening the stomach muscles. Both should be done with the knees bent, so as not to strain the back. Sit-ups are done with the arms behind the head, curl-ups with the arms crossed over the abdomen. During both exercises, the pelvis should be tilted, pressing the small of the back into the supporting surface. For a sit-up, the torso should be brought to the sitting position; for a curl-up, the head and shoulders should be curled up until the shoulder blades have cleared the floor and the position held for a moment. Starting with as many repetitions as can be performed easily, you should gradually increase the exercise until a maximum of 50 to 100 (depending on your age) can be accomplished during one exercise period.

Q: Do all people benefit from Williams' exercises, which flex the back (bend it forward)?

A: No. Ten percent to twenty percent of people with back problems get more relief from exercises that extend rather than flex the back (Mackenzie exercises). These exercises involve lying flat on your stomach and arching your back by pressing up with your arms. People also test various motions to see which position can "centralize" their pain, causing it to retreat toward the midline.

Q: Is a waterbed harmful for someone with back pain?

A: Usually, but not necessarily. As mentioned, the best sleeping surface for most sufferers of back pain is an extra-firm mattress. However, a few people seem to be more comfortable on a waterbed. If you are one of them, by all means continue to use the type of bed that provides the most comfort.

Q: How do I know when my back is bad enough for me to go to my doctor?

A: It is certainly time to seek expert medical attention:
   (1) when you have tried home remedies for a few days and you are either not getting better or getting worse;
   (2) when the pain is severe enough to keep you up at night and away from work;
   (3) when you have pain or numbness radiating into your legs; or
   (4) when you have weakness in your legs or notice any difficulty urinating or moving your bowels.

Other clues to a more serious illness causing back pain are unexplained weight loss, substantial trauma, point tenderness in the back, a history of cancer or osteoporosis, risk factors for vascular disease (smoking, high cholesterol, and so on), chronic use of steroids, and inability to find a comfortable position.

Q: How many vertebrae are there in the back?

A: There are seven cervical (neck) vertebrae, twelve thoracic (chest) vertebrae, five lumbar (low back) vertebrae, plus the sacrum and the coccyx (tailbone). Sometimes the upper segment of the sacrum remains as a separate vertebra, and occasionally the fifth lumbar vertebra fuses to the sacrum. The coccyx is a vestigial tail, and a child may be born with a coccygeal stump that hearkens back to an arboreal ancestor, but this is rare.

10

The Neck

A mole on the neck, you shall have money by the peck

Old English Rhyme

The neck is one of the first places in which pain occurs as the result of stress. It is no coincidence that people often somaticize tension to the neck—our organ language reflects this in the common complaint, "He/she is a pain in the neck." Because the neck is the gateway, as it were, to the shoulders and arms in one direction and the head in the other direction, difficulties that originate in the neck can result in symptoms such as headache (usually in the rear or occipital area), dizziness or nausea, pain or cramping in the arms, and tingling or numbness in the fingers.

The neck is a pathway that carries the spinal cord as well as crucial nerves and blood vessels to the rest of the body. The head may weigh more than 20 pounds and is entirely supported by the neck. The neck is therefore very vulnerable to pain or injury, and this vulnerability is increased by its mobility.

Seven stacked bones called *cervical vertebrae* comprise the bony structure of the neck (Figure 10-1). Movement of these vertebrae is controlled by a variety of muscles, which are held in place by numerous ligaments. The major arteries to the head are carried through the neck, and the spinal nerves that serve the arms leave the spinal cord between these vertebrae.

Like the vertebrae of the back, the neck vertebrae are separated by pads of fibrous cartilage, called *discs,* which act as shock absorbers. Also like the vertebrae of the back, those of

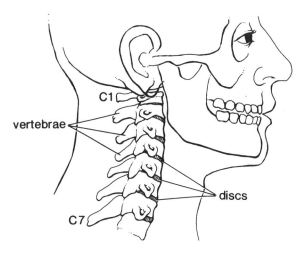

FIGURE 10-1   The Cervical Spine

the neck contain joints (facets) that permit significant motion, including 180 degrees of rotation, approximately 120 degrees of tilt to either side, and almost 90 degrees of forward (flexion) and backward (extension) bending. Most mammals have the same seven neck bones as we do, even the giraffe, whose neck can reach over six feet in length. Elongation of the neck is considered a sign of female beauty and status by some African tribes. This is accomplished by stacking metal rings on a native girl's neck during growth. In this way, the neck is not lengthened so much as the girl's shoulders are depressed, giving the appearance of elongation, sometimes by 50 percent or more.

The cervical vertebrae are numbered 1 to 7, starting with the one closest to the skull. C1 is called the atlas, C2 the axis. These names are conferred because the first cervical vertebra literally (like Atlas) supports the head, and through its special design C2 enables axial rotation of approximately 180 degrees of the head on the neck.

In addition to tension, neck pain can occur from chronic malposture, arthritis (either osteoarthritis or inflammatory arthritis), any disease process that can involve bone (tumor, infection, and so forth), or accidents that cause sprains and strains. More serious injuries include fractures or dislocations, which frequently occur during athletic contact, industrial mishaps, or automobile collisions.

The common "whiplash" injury usually occurs when a standing automobile is struck from behind or an accelerating vehicle hits a solid object. In either case, because of the sudden impact, the head keeps moving and as it passes over the stationary neck, in either hyperextension (backwards) or hyperflexion (forwards), the vertebrae are compressed. This causes the neck to accept a force of well over 500 pounds. This may result in ligamentous and bony damage. Discomfort includes pain, which can be referred to the shoulder or arm, as well as headache, nausea, dizziness (which may be secondary to injury to the blood vessels), and persistent neck stiffness.

Most whiplash injuries, like other sprains, respond to conservative treatment, including moist heat, cervical traction (either intermittent or continuous), the use of an appropriate myocervical collar support, special cervical pillows, diathermy and massage, a TENS unit, and appropriate anti-pain medication (anodynes) or nonsteroidal anti-inflammatory drugs (NSAIDs).

POSTURE

Because the spine is like the axle of a vehicle, it cannot be malaligned at one end without causing trouble at the other end. Proper posture is very important to ensure not only a healthy back but also a healthy and pain-free neck. Any job or hobby that requires a lot of leaning tends to stress the neck. Frequent relief of this strain by changing position and using neck stretching and strengthening exercises will go a long way toward preventing common neck problems secondary to postural malalignment or emotional tension.

NECK STRETCHING EXERCISES

1. Sit well back in straight back chair, feet hooked inside around front chair legs.
2. Rotate head, neck, and body to the right as far as possible.
3. Bring left arm across chest and grasp chair along right side of body.
4. Place palm of right hand around left side of tip of closed jaw.

5. Now pull with left arm and push jaw with right hand at the same time as much as can be tolerated.

6. Do this for ten seconds and then relax. Repeat five times.

7. Now rotate to the left, reverse arms, and stretch neck to the left as above.

8. Do these exercises three times each day.

ISOMETRIC EXERCISES FOR THE NECK

These exercises can strengthen the neck. They are particularly useful for someone weaning himself from a neck collar.

The head moves in six directions on the neck: (1) forward, (2) backward, (3) tilting to the right, (4) tilting to the left, (5) rotating to the right, and (6) rotating to the left.

Restraining motion of the head by linking the hands and placing them on the forehead, attempt to move the head by forcing it against the hands to a slow count of six. Relax.

Now place the linked hands behind the head and repeat the exercise attempting to force the head backwards. Remember to use maximum strength to a slow count of six. Relax.

Use the right hand to restrain the head from tilting to the right as you repeat the exercise as above.

Now use the left hand, blocking a forceful attempt to tilt the head to the left. Remember to use maximum strength to a slow count of six. Relax.

Finally, restrain rotation to the right by cupping the right hand under the chin. Forcefully attempt to rotate the head to the right again to a slow count of six. Relax.

Repeat the attempt to rotate the head and neck, this time to the left while using the left hand cupped under the left side of the chin as a restraint.

Remember, these are isometric exercises that rely on a forceful muscle contraction. You must exert at least 75 percent of maximal muscle force for any benefit. The head and neck must be kept in line and upright facing forward and should not move during the exercise. This training regimen is designed to strengthen all the muscles of the neck. The entire exercise program takes less than one minute. It should be performed three times a day.

Wear and tear processes, such as those found in arthritic joints, can affect the bones and joints of the neck. These typically occur in areas at which most motion in the neck occurs, usually at the level of the fourth through sixth cervical vertebrae. Arthritis or disc disease in the neck may require treatment similar to that for arthritis elsewhere in the body. This includes the occasional necessity for operations such as fusion (stabilization) of several vertebrae or decompression (relief of pressure) by removing bone and/or a protruding or herniated disc that is pinching a nerve.

Any neck problem that does not readily respond to simple conservative home treatment should be referred to your doctor, who will take a history and perform a physical examination, including a thorough neurologic study of the head, neck, shoulders, and arms. X-rays and occasionally a blood test may be ordered. Special tests, including CT scans and MRI examinations, EMG, and NCV, also help to decide whether or not pressure on a nerve is playing a role in pain causation.

SEVEN RULES TO KEEP YOUR NECK IN SHAPE

1. Do not strain your neck. Avoid craning and sudden neck motions, particularly looking high overhead or twisting the neck. To prevent strain, avoid forward thrust ("spectator's attitude") positions of the head and neck.
2. Use a firm, level sleeping surface. A small pillow is preferable to keep head level with the rest of the body.
3. A chair that has a high back and arm supports will relieve neck muscle tension.
4. Apply some heat (hot shower, hot towel, hot moist compress, heating pad on low) to your neck at least twice daily.
5. A large bath towel, rolled or folded lengthwise and wrapped about the neck, will provide gentle support and warmth.
6. Nightly massage with cold cream or balm relaxes muscles and increases circulation.
7. Life situations that provoke grief, resentment, guilt, anger, or other negative emotional responses may initiate or aggravate nervous and muscular tension states.

After determining the specific cause of your problem, your doctor will advise a neck care program tailored to your needs. This may include frequent periods of rest with a special supportive neck pillow. A soft or firm cervical collar may be prescribed. Home traction is another simple method of relieving pressure by taking the strain off the neck muscles. This is typically applied with the neck in slight flexion with the chin tilted forward, the position in which a sufferer of neck pain should learn to carry his neck. Acute muscle spasm is usually relieved by ice, whereas chronic pain or spasm often respond to moist heat (shower, bath, hot water bottle, hot compress, moist heating pad). Injections of local anesthetic or cortisone into trigger pain areas can often break the vicious cycle of pain and muscle spasm that occurs with chronic neck problems. Massage can help, as well as exercises that stretch the neck muscles.

Physical therapy is a more formal way of applying these treatments. The therapist may apply heat using moist hot packs or deep electrical diathermy and may administer intermittent traction with a motorized unit. The patient is instructed in appropriate range of motion exercises to increase neck mobility and isometric workouts to increase strength. An occupational therapist will review the patient's lifestyle and methods for handling tasks of daily living and can then recommend ways and means to avoid neck strain on the job and at home.

The thing to remember is that you do not have to put up with neck tension and pain. By following a program that includes relaxation, proper posture, increasing range of motion, and strengthening of your neck, you can develop a balanced neck and avoid the recurrent stiffness and pain that accompany the neglected neck syndrome.

Let's shift gears now and visit the most frequently abused joint in the body, the knee.

QUESTIONS AND ANSWERS ABOUT THE NECK

Q: What is torticollis?

A: Literally, a twisted neck (*torque*, to twist; *collum*, neck—both from the Latin), a wry neck. This can be caused by any number of conditions, some serious, most not. The common stiff neck occurs from sleeping in an awkward position, exposing the neck to an unusual temperature change (such as direct air conditioning), or sustaining a sudden twist or jar. The best remedy is icing followed by heat and rest with stretching and isometric exercises.

Q: Is there a normal curve to the cervical vertebrae?

A: Yes, and it is a lordotic curve, similar to that of the lumbar spine. Straightening of this curve can indicate muscle spasm secondary to pathology in the neck.

Q: Are "slipped discs" as common in the neck as they are in the low back?

A: No, they are not. The anatomy of the cervical vertebrae is such that the edge of the bone curves slightly, producing a restraining barrier to protrusion of the disc. Also, the cervical vertebrae are not commonly subjected to the magnitude of forces that load the lumbar spine.

Q: How can one avoid straining the neck during daily activity?

A: This may be impossible but some suggestions are (1) use a straw rather than drink from a bottle; (2) do not tilt your head back when shaving or washing; (3) use a shower instead of washing your hair in a sink; (4) use a head rest to support your head while driving; (5) avoid prolonged riding or driving, and make regular stops to rest; (6) take frequent breaks during work and leisure activities; (7) try not to sleep on your stomach; it is better for your neck to sleep on your side or back.

11

The Knee

Ministering angels have no knees
as they must always stand in the presence of God.

Commentary to the Orthodox Hebrew Prayer Book

The knee is the largest of the 187 joints in the body. It is subject to a variety of diseases and is frequently injured because it is often abused. The human knee was not designed to withstand the excessive strain that is often placed on it, particularly by weekend athletes. Almost half a million knee operations are performed yearly in the United States. Nearly 70 percent of all football players will have knee surgery by the time they are 26 years old. Damage to the ligaments of the knee is the most common ski injury, and it occurs more frequently in the recreational basketball player than all other injuries combined. Knee disorders are the number one reason why people visit orthopaedic surgeons.

Our knees tell us they are in trouble when they are painful, swell (this can be due to an accumulation of fluid or blood within the knee), become stiff (nature's way of splinting a joint), lock, or give way. Any of these signs or symptoms can be acute (sudden) or chronic (long-standing). The knee is very vulnerable to sprains or strains. Simply walking up stairs places at least three times your body weight on the knee at each step, and descending stairs subjects the knee (as well as the hip) to seven times your weight! That is why the cartilage that covers the knee must be thicker than anywhere else in the body. Arthritis, both inflammatory and degenerative, can affect the knee as a weight-bearing joint.

The knee is surrounded by a number of bursae that may become inflamed and swollen (Figure 11-1). One common bursitis about the knee is the so-called *housemaid's knee,* which occurs in the bursal sac that lies just in front of the patella (kneecap). A similar bursitis in the back of the knee is called a Baker's cyst (after the man who first described it, not the trade). Like any joint, the knee can be fractured, ligaments may be torn, and, with severe force, the knee joint may even dislocate. (This usually occurs during water skiing, water being a noncompressible substance.) Various deformities of the knees are seen during childhood. Knock-knee and bowleg are usually self-limited, but may persist into adolescence and require surgical correction.

The knee is essentially a hinged joint although it has some rotation to provide locking. Two cartilage pads separate the knee bones, the *semilunar cartilages* or *menisci* (Greek: *meniskos,* meaning a crescent moon), which provide cushioning and a shock absorber effect. These cartilages are frequently injured, especially the inside or medial one, and particularly in sports that require cutting and twisting.

Four major ligaments stabilize the knee. The two collateral ligaments bind the femur to the tibia medially and laterally (inside and outside), and two *cruciate ligaments*—called so because they cross inside the joint—traverse the interior of the knee. Knee ligaments are prone to stretching and tearing

FIGURE 11-1   Your Knee Anatomy

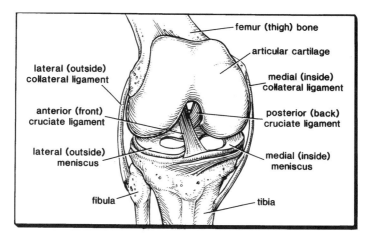

during injuries, especially the medial collateral and anterior (front) cruciate ligaments. An example of this is breaststroker's knee, found in competitive swimmers, a stress injury to the inside of the knee incurred during the breaststroke kick. In more violent injuries such as those that occur in football, it is not uncommon to have tears of the medial meniscus associated with rupture of both the medial collateral and anterior cruciate ligaments. This is called the "terrible triad."

The large muscles of the thigh provide strength and stability to the knee, particularly the quadriceps muscle group in the front and the hamstrings in the back. The quadriceps has four (L. quadri-) heads or parts (L. caput). The hamstrings are the five muscles whose tendons are severed when an animal such as a bull is hamstrung in order to cripple it. These muscles weaken and waste rapidly after knee injury. Maintaining muscle tone is important in the prevention of injury as well as in rehabilitation after injury or surgery. Disuse atrophy (wasting) due to immobilization of the knee, for whatever reason, can delay recovery. After all, it is the medial (inside) portion of the quadriceps that allows people to attain their upright posture. Apes lack this muscle and therefore walk in a crouched posture. This is the first muscle to waste after injury, making it difficult to walk upright. Therefore, exercising is very important to maintain healthy knees. However, some exercises, particularly knee squats, place a great deal of strain on the cruciate ligaments and should be avoided. The maximum force across the knee occurs at 35 degrees of flexion. This means that more than seven times body weight is being transmitted to the knee during a deep knee bend. It is better to use isometric exercises, engage in resistance exercising, or bike or swim.

DIAGNOSING AND TREATING KNEE PROBLEMS

The diagnosis of a knee disorder is no different from the diagnosis of a problem in any other joint. A history will be taken and a physical examination performed. If the knee is swollen, it may be aspirated and the fluid analyzed for cells and crystals, such as those found in gout or a related condition called pseudogout. An x-ray will no doubt be ordered. X-rays taken with the knee under stress may be necessary to diagnose instability due to ligamentous laxity. There are also special x-ray techniques such as arthrography, in which a water-soluble dye is injected and x-rays performed. This helps visualize tears in the menisci. CT scans and MRI examinations as well as bone scans may also be ordered.

Diagnostic arthroscopy is frequently used in the management of knee problems. Many famous knees have been arthroscoped. Mikhail Baryshnikov had his looked into twice! This procedure is usually carried out in a hospital operating room or an outpatient surgicenter. General anesthesia may be required, although arthroscopy can be performed with a local anesthetic. Most arthroscopic procedures are done on an outpatient basis and do not call for an overnight stay in the hospital.

QUADRICEPS STRENGTHENING KNEE MUSCLE EXERCISES

1. Lie on your back on a firm, flat surface, keeping your knee perfectly straight and stiff (180 degrees). Lift the leg as high as possible. Slowly return the leg to the resting position. Relax momentarily.

During this exercise, tension should be felt in the muscles of the front of the thigh. Do as many straight leg lifts as possible the first day. Gradually increase the number you can perform by adding one repetition each succeeding day to a maximum of fifty lifts. Continue with fifty lifts daily. Proceed slowly; you may feel fatigued but should not experience pain.

2. Comfortably seated with a shoe on, hook the foot of the involved knee under a desk, sofa, chair, or other piece of furniture too heavy to lift. Keeping the knee perfectly straight and stiff, attempt to lift the furniture, exerting a maximal effort and slowly counting to six. Relax. During the exercise, tension should be felt in the muscles of the front of the thigh. Next, bend the knee approximately 30 degrees, and repeat the exercise. Finally, bend the knee approximately 60 degrees, and repeat again.

These are isometric exercises. The knee should not move during the six-second maximal contracture. Each exercise is to be performed only once during an exercise period. Repeat these isometric exercises three times a day.

In addition to diagnosis, surgery can be performed through the arthroscope using specially designed instruments. Loose bony and cartilaginous fragments can be removed, portions of torn cartilage excised, damaged joint surfaces repaired, meniscal tears sutured, ligaments mended, and biopsies taken. Occasionally the necessary surgical repair may be extensive enough to require opening the knee. This is usually done at the same time as the diagnostic arthroscopy in order to avoid an additional anesthetic. Incidentally, both diagnostic and surgical arthroscopy can also be performed on other joints, including the shoulder, elbow, hip, wrist, and ankle.

Recovery after knee surgery, arthroscopic or otherwise, involves guarded weight bearing. This may require the temporary use of crutches or a cane, rest with ice packs initially, and rehabilitation exercises. A cast or brace may sometimes be necessary. A variety of braces have also been proposed to *prevent* knee injury, particularly in football quarterbacks, but whether the research takes place in a laboratory or on the playing field, the effectiveness of such bracing remains inconclusive.

It is important to understand that, although knee arthroscopy accounts for at least 90 percent of all knee surgery today, in the proper hands it is diagnostically close to 100 percent accurate. Such super-athletes as gymnast Mary Lou Retton and marathoner Joan Benoit underwent arthroscopy just before qualifying for the 1984 Olympic games. However, arthroscopy is still surgery and has a complication rate of up to 15 percent, including postoperative bleeding, damage to articular cartilage, and even instrument breakage in the joint during the procedure.

Other than the conditions already mentioned, some of the most common knee problems include an unstable or dislocating patella, usually at the outside of the knee. This may be caused by injury, although people with knock-knee are prone to having their kneecaps slip out of place. Such instability can sometimes be remedied by appropriate exercises and wearing an elastic or neoprene knee support (Palumbo style knee sleeve) during athletics. Occasionally an operation designed to align the kneecap in its groove may be indicated.

Roughening of the articular cartilage of the patella is called *chondromalacia* (cartilage softening). This leads to irritation, with swelling and pain. The patient may experience crepitation (grinding) on knee motion, and pain often occurs after prolonged sitting with the knee bent. Chondromalacia is frequently seen in teenagers during rapid spurts of growth. It is more common in girls and may be related to hormonal change in adolescence. It is treated with anti-inflammatory medications, quadriceps strengthening exercises, and the use of light elastic knee supports. Occasionally, arthroscopic surgery is necessary to smooth the roughened cartilage and, rarely, an operation must be performed to reposition or remove the patella.

Areas of growing cartilage may become inflamed during periods of rapid growth. One such area is found in the front of the tibia at the knee joint. An exquisitely painful bump may develop. This is called Osgood-Schlatter's disease, immortalizing the two physicians who first described the condition. It is most frequently found in boys during puberty who apparently stress their knees more often than girls. Treatment consists of rest, icing, pain medication, avoiding bumping the knee by using a padded knee guard, and occasionally by using a protective plaster cast for a brief period of time. The condition is self-limited but will not entirely resolve until growth is complete, which may take several years. The patient is left with a bump in front of his knee, which is no problem unless he enters a profession that requires frequent kneeling, such as the priesthood.

Osteochondritis (bone-cartilage inflammation) *dissecans* (to separate) is a condition, usually found in children, in which a small piece of articular cartilage separates because its underlying bone dies; this often occurs on the femoral (upper) side of the knee joint. This condition is thought to be caused by repeated minor trauma. The cartilage-bony fragment may break off and float around as a loose body or "joint mouse" in the knee. If the fragment has not separated, treatment is to restrict activity. Once separation has started, arthroscopic surgery is necessary to either remove the fragment or to pin it back into place.

Your knees will serve you long and well if you take care of them with proper exercise, avoid abusing them, and seek medical treatment when necessary. If an operation is required, do not despair. Remember that such well-known athletes as Joe Montana and Magic Johnson had knee surgery and continued to play afterwards.

Next, let's visit another set of nearby joints, the foot.

QUESTIONS AND ANSWERS ABOUT THE KNEE

Q: Are women's knees more at risk for injury then men's?
A: Some say yes. The characteristics of the female body contribute to this vulnerability. Women may be more disposed to knee injury because their wider hips cause the femur to turn inward, putting more pressure on their knees. The extra width at the hips also contributes to knock-knees. Finally,

women have 20 percent less muscle mass than men, so pound for pound there is less muscle to support the knee.

Q: What are pathologic synovial plicae?

A: Synovial plicae are portions of thin, membranous walls that separated the three knee compartments during development. These developmental left-overs are found in up to 50 percent of normal knees. Sometimes these bands, like adhesions in the abdomen, can cause acute or chronic knee pain. If conservative treatment, including rest and medication, fail to bring relief, arthroscopic release or removal of these annoying plicae is usually successful.

Q: Is it necessary to remove the entire meniscus when only part of it is torn?

A: It is not only unnecessary but undesirable, because the meniscus protects the knee from developing osteoarthritis. More than 90 percent of the 100,000 or so meniscectomies done yearly in the United States are only partial. Additionally, if the tear is along the margin of the meniscus where blood supply is adequate, it can often be sewn up and will heal.

Q: What is the "terrible triad" injury?

A: The "terrible triad" injury occurs in an athlete who receives a blow to the outside of his knee while the foot is planted and the knee bent. In such a situation, the medial meniscus can be crushed in the knee and the anterior cruciate may give way. As force continues, the medial collateral ligament also stretches or tears. This is why "clipping" is a serious penalty in football.

Q: Some sports medicine centers use a Cybex machine. What is this?

A: A Cybex machine is an apparatus that matches a patient's resistance during exercise. It can measure range of motion, power, endurance, and strength. These capabilities are recorded by a computer and the resulting print-out used to keep track of a patient's rehabilitation. The Cybex can also reveal otherwise unrecognized muscle weakness. Thus, a customized muscle strengthening program can be prescribed.

Q: Is it always necessary to surgically repair torn ligaments in the knee?

A: No. Often immobilizing the knee in an appropriate cast or brace will allow a torn collateral ligament to heal as well or even better than if it had been repaired surgically. In the case of the anterior cruciate ligament, its absence can leave very of the anterior cruciate ligament, its absence can leave very little instability or functional disability.

A strong quadriceps muscle can often compensate for a torn anterior cruciate and, except in cases of top-notch professional athletes who require "Cadillac" knees, the absence of this ligament does not preclude modest recreational athletics. Repair can be difficult and must be supplemented with other natural tendon such as a slip from the patellar tendon or an artificial ligament made of a carbon composite. Rehabilitation may be prolonged and involved, often taking as long as a year and requiring a brace. Although it can usually be accomplished through an arthroscope, reconstruction of a torn anterior cruciate ligament is not a procedure to be taken lightly.

Q: Is rehabilitation necessary after knee surgery?

A: Absolutely! Surgery is useless without rehabilitation. This involves specific rehabilitative exercises, starting with quadriceps drill without weights and progressing to weights as tolerated.

Even without surgery, braces that provide immobility to facilitate soft tissue repair and exercises that stimulate muscle strengthening are prescribed. Rehabilitation can be divided into three phases. First is the phase of rest, second is that of exercise to rebuild strength and endurance, and last is conditioning for full functional performance.

Special techniques of rehabilitation include water work-outs that involve exercising in a pool to take advantage of both the buoyancy provided to an injured limb as well as the resistance provided by the water.

Q: Are different types of exercises used in rehabilitating an injured knee?

A: Yes. Range of motion exercises are used to help regain full joint movement; strengthening exercises increase power; functional exercises recover useful movements; and stretching exercises stretch out contractures. Aerobic exercise increases flexibility and endurance.

Q: What is the Lenox-Hill brace?

A: The Lenox-Hill brace is a custom-made appliance that was popularized in 1969 by the New York Jets quarterback, Joe Namath. It is a derotation appliance that weighs less than two pounds and has seven straps that support the knee externally in the same way it should normally be supported by intact ligaments. The brace may cost as much as $1,000, but if you need one, it is well worth it.

Q: Some people have a kneecap removed. How is it possible to function without the kneecap?

A: Sometimes the patella has to be removed because it is shattered or severely arthritic. The knee can function reasonably well without a kneecap. However, because the kneecap acts as a pulley for quadriceps muscle action, in its absence the quadriceps tendon falls back onto the joint, and the muscle must be at least 30 percent stronger in order to stabilize the knee as well as it did before removal of the kneecap.

Q: Which meniscus is torn most frequently?

A: The medial (inside) meniscus is more frequently torn because it is larger, more mobile, and more vulnerable. The lateral (outer) meniscus can also be torn. Wrestlers are more likely to suffer lateral tears.

Because more than 70 percent of the meniscus is without a blood supply, healing is very poor. The only meniscal tears that lend themselves to repair rather than excision are those of the outer margin, where the blood supply is more plentiful. Incidentally, once a meniscus is removed, nothing like the original cartilage will grow back in its place.

12

A Foot User's Guide

Keep your mouth wet and your feet dry.

Benjamin Franklin
Poor Richard's Almanac, 1733

The entire task of balancing the body during standing and walking takes place on an area that measures only a few square inches, the soles of the feet. And not even the entire soles, because approximately one-third of the foot does not touch the ground but instead is curved upward to create an arch that minimizes the shock taken with each step.

How wonderful our feet are! Both together absorb more than 700 tons of force a day. In a lifetime, in walking 1.2×10^6 steps each year, they can carry an average person almost 75,000 miles, or approximately three times around the Earth's equator. It is claimed that a man walks approximately six miles a day, a woman about nine. The average pedestrian exerts approximately 450 pounds of pressure on the feet with each step taken.

Bipedal (two-footed) ambulation is seen only in primates and reaches its greatest sophistication in us. The process of developing our pattern of walking began several million years ago, freeing our arms and hands for creative tasks. Foot care was judged to be very important even in biblical times. The plantar arch was mentioned in the Old Testament, in which reference to foot care, particularly washing of the feet, is made at least four times in the book of Genesis. Apparently the ancient Israelites had healthy feet, since no edema (swelling) was reported during their 40 years of wandering in the Sinai. ". . . Neither did thy foot swell, these forty years." But *your* feet may swell from time to time. The heart is not the only organ in the body that acts as a pump; so do the leg muscles. Walking assists the pumping effect. Prolonged inactivity, such as sitting on an airplane (particularly with the legs crossed), causes blood and other fluids to collect in the feet with the assistance of gravity. The remedy is to avoid sitting for prolonged periods whether on a plane, train, bus, or even in an office. Get up and move around frequently, so that your leg muscles have a chance to pump and keep your feet from swelling.

Simple sandals were the first footwear, although in ancient Rome only the aristocracy were permitted sandals; slaves went barefoot. Shoes have served cosmetic as well as functional roles throughout history. Early actors used platform shoes to elevate characters on stage. Chinese women bound their feet as a sign of well-bred beauty. This started with the Chinese Empress Ta-Ki (1100 A.D.) whose club foot prompted a royal edict that all women's feet should look like those of their Empress. The custom left many otherwise exquisite women with severely deformed feet and a permanent limp. In medieval times pointed shoes were thought to keep witches away. It was not until after the Civil War that American shoes were designed with a separate right and left last. It is well known that Abraham Lincoln had custom shoes made because of his problem with bunions. Lincoln employed a podiatrist on a regular basis—who, incidentally, also acted as a spy for the North.

Feet have long been a sexual symbol. Toe-kissing is a part of lovemaking in India. Alfred Kinsey reports that the toes curl or spread during sexual arousal. No wonder foot fetishes abound.

The modern woman is faced with a fashionable assault on the integrity of her feet through the use of narrow pointed toes and high heels. These were first introduced by Catherine de Medici (1519–1589) of France. Ordinary weight bearing places 40 percent of the weight on the toes and 60 percent on the heel. This can be reversed when the heel is elevated. You can imagine the pain and problems a woman can get into when cramping her toes so loaded into a narrow pointed shoe. In fact the little toe of today is smaller than it was a century ago because of all this squeezing. Animal feet also reflect adaptive changes. The original horse had four toes on each foot, whereas the modern equus has only one, the hoof being its toenail. Men also are not immune from foot problems, particularly if they have inherited wide feet or high arches. Although their shoes are usually roomier and more comfortable, men tend to abuse their feet through overweight and stress, particularly with occasional athletic activity. Honest Abe said, "when my feet hurt, I can't think." Apparently he was not alone. Last year alone, more than $200 million was spent on proprietary remedies for the relief of foot complaints.

This chapter explains how your foot is constructed and how it helps you perform tasks that require standing and walking. It illustrates some of the common problems that foot owners can encounter and how they are prevented and treated. Finally, you should learn how to take care of your feet so they can stand up for you when you need them.

UNDERSTANDING YOUR FEET

Each foot has 26 bones, constructed to form two arches (Figure 12-1). The *long arch* is located at the instep and the *transverse* (metatarsal) *arch* runs across the ball of the foot. These arches act as shock absorbers and tend to flatten on weight bearing. Some people are "flatfooted," but this is usually not a severe disability. Many great athletes have been flatfooted, and cultures such as the American Indian, whose soft moccasins offered foot protection but minimal support, were habitually flatfooted. Yet they were able to run, climb, and track with amazing agility. Children up to the age of three or four years do not display a long arch because this area is filled with baby fat. Adolescent girls who have functionally flat feet will develop an arch when they begin wearing a higher heeled shoe. The only serious type of flat foot is the spastic type, which is accompanied by a congenital fusion of several bones in the mid- or hindfoot. High, rigid arches are usually more painful than flat ones and, in fact, may be indicative of a more general neuromuscular disorder. Flattening of the long arch may also be due to a tight heel cord. Dropping of the transverse arch can occur secondary to other conditions, which will be discussed later.

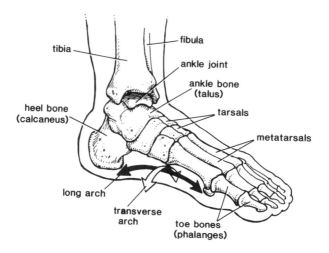

FIGURE 12-1   Anatomy of the Foot

There are 33 joints in the foot, which keep it flexible. Foot movement is controlled by 38 muscles, originating both within and without the foot proper. The bones of the foot are held together by 56 ligaments, many of which may be strained or sprained during a twist or fall.

Infants first learning to walk tend to waddle, throwing their feet out (out-toeing) in order to increase the width of their base of support and prevent falling. This condition, as well as the occasional pigeon-toeing (in-toeing), tends to resolve as the child gains balance with growth. Mild knock-knees or bowlegs are also reflections of early incoordination and do the same.

The feet are amazing locomotor organs. Leonardo da Vinci claimed them "a masterpiece of engineering and a work of art." Walking can best be described as a controlled fall. You lose balance, gain balance, lose balance, gain balance, over and over again. Your feet monitor rather than motivate ambulation. Most of the metabolic energy expended by the feet during walking is used to slow gait and keep the body from completely falling. To do this, each foot must step much like a jet airplane lands, that is, with the wheels (heel) down and the nose (toes) up. Therefore, each step is a heel-toe rhythm with takeoff on your toes and full weight bearing on each foot alternately as the other swings through. On *stance*, weight is borne on the tripod of the heel, the base of the great toe, and the base of the fifth toe. Body weight is centered over the feet, the inner borders remaining rigid for support and the outer flexible to adapt to variations in contour of the walking surface.

IF THE SHOE FITS . . .

If the shoe fits, wear it! And if it doesn't, don't! Poorly fitting shoes can lead to a wide variety of problems. It has been said that "if you want to forget your troubles, wear a pair of tight shoes!"

A good shoe should have a firm sole and a light upper. The insole is best if it is cushioned, and although any size heel can be used for a brief period of time, regularly worn heels should be of low or medium height. If you cannot touch your toes, your calf muscles are tight and you will be more comfortable in a higher heel. If you can, a flatter shoe is more appropriate. The counter of the shoe must fit snugly so that the instep does not gape. There must be adequate toe room, and the toe box should be wide enough to accommodate the forefoot. The second toe is the longest in approximately 20 percent of people. This must be taken into account during fitting. The vamp of the shoe should be high enough to provide adequate support.

Because foot size and shape may change with age, it is wise to have your feet measured each time you buy new shoes. Both feet should be measured because they may be different sizes, and shoes should be purchased for the larger foot. The largest men's shoes ever sold were worn by Harley Davidson of Avon Park, Florida. His feet were size 42; that is the equivalent of five size 8 1/2 shoes placed end to end. It is best to go shopping for shoes later in the day because feet tend to swell at that time. The shoes you buy must be comfortable enough to wear from the store—do not buy uncomfortable shoes intending to "break them in." For senior citizens, athletic shoes with plush, spongy soles are the worst kind for maintaining balance and can lead to falls. With a thick cushiony shoe, it is more difficult to judge the angle of your foot in relation to the ground. For older people a shoe such as a boating shoe or topsider, with a relatively thin, hard rubber sole, is better for maintaining balance.

Lasts are the three-dimensional forms over which shoes are made. The lasts used for women's athletic shoes are often smaller versions of men's shoes, ignoring the anatomic shape of a woman's foot. These inconsistencies can cause injuries to the female athlete's feet, including aggravation of bunions, corns, calluses, hammertoes, pinched nerves, and toenail avulsion. Before the 1980s, the only sport shoe specifically designed to the anatomic shape of a woman's foot was for golf. Women have a different gait than men because they have a wider pelvis, a different angle to the hip, more knock-knee, and more flatness of their hindfeet. These factors help keep the plumb line of the body centered. Additionally, women have narrower heels and shorter legs relative to their height. Competitive female runners are predominantly midfoot strikers as compared with male heel strikers. They also strike the ground more often for the same distance, generating more ground reaction forces.

Even though women spend more on athletic shoes than men, many manufacturers continue to make shoes for women that are basically designed for men's feet. Consumers should be educated to these facts and understand that shoes can be built of either a slip last (lightweight and flexible), a board last (rigid and stable), or a combination last (forefoot flexibility and heel stability) for a customized fit. Athletic shoes should be purchased just before sport participation, when the feet are largest. The runner should run some in the shoe store wearing the same socks that will be worn during the race, and test the shoes on an incline for slipping.

A proper fit can be fine-tuned by varying the lacing techniques as indicated. For instance, in shoes with a double set of eyelets bordering the tongue, a narrow foot can be accommodated by lacing the widest set of eyelets to tighten the shoe away from the foot. For wide feet, lace the eyelets closest to the tongue for more width in the lacing area. Leave a gap in the laces over any bony prominence or point of pressure pain.

Concerning children's shoes, shoes are more for protection than support until a child begins to spend most of his time on his feet (after about 18 months), and the lightest possible footwear should be used. A well-fitted leather oxford is usually best unless a child has a particular problem that requires special shoes or shoe adaptations (wedges, inserts, a special last). High-topped shoes do not offer additional support for a normal foot, although admittedly they may be more difficult for a child to remove. Children's shoes should be checked frequently as the feet grow in spurts and cramping can easily occur. Used shoes should not be passed down from one child to another.

BE NICE TO YOUR FEET

It stands to reason that if you are nice to your feet, they will be nice to you. If you have ever had painful feet, you know that this is one of the most pervasive complaints you can suffer. Following some simple rules of foot care can keep your feet fit for the next step. Nails should be trimmed straight across to avoid the corners cutting into the flesh and causing ingrown nails. The feet should be washed daily, dried thoroughly, and a mild medicated foot powder used. Stockings must fit, and they should be changed daily. Feet that tend to perspire more than usual can benefit from wearing leather or canvas shoes or sandals, with frequent switching of footwear. The average adult foot perspires one-eighth pint of moisture a day. Dark hose trap heat and increase perspiration. Porous insoles help air get to the foot.

William Scholl, the Chicago shoemaker and shoe salesman who attended night school to become a doctor, recommended wearing two pairs of shoes a day, so each pair could dry out. Dr. Scholl created a national foot consciousness to which he catered with his familiar yellow-and-blue packaged foot aids. Scholl, who died in 1968 at age 86, boasted that he never forgot a foot.

The elderly must be particularly careful about their feet, as should individuals who have poor foot circulation or diseases such as diabetes. They need to avoid any rubbing that could cause a blister leading to an ulcer or infection, which in turn might require surgery, even an amputation. Because their feet may have diminished sensation, they must be checked several times each day for any abrasions or irritations. Constricting stockings or shoes should be avoided. The feet should not be exposed to excessive heat or cold, even inadvertently. A doctor must be consulted immediately for any foot pain, discoloration, or evidence of even minimal disease.

A note about proprietary foot care. Self-treatment may be harmful. It is unwise to use over-the-counter medications to treat corns or calluses because many such preparations have an acid base that can irritate the feet. Some foot problems reflect a more general state of disease, so when in doubt it is best to seek professional advice for specific diagnosis and treatment.

COMMON FOOT PROBLEMS

Ingrown Toenails

Onychocryptosis (hidden nail) is the medical term for an ingrown toenail. This condition occurs when the nail grows into the skin next to it, causing inflammation and sometimes overt infection. This most commonly happens along the inside border of the great toenails. Few people can escape at least one ingrown toenail in a lifetime. The most common causes of ingrown toenails are pressure on the toenail from poorly fitting socks or shoes or improper trimming of the nail. A fungus infection, which can produce thickening, darkening, brittleness, and curving of the nail, can cause or aggravate ingrown toenails.

By far the major cause of ingrown toenails is improper nail trimming. Whereas fingernails should be trimmed in a curved fashion, toenails should be cut straight across, leaving the outer nail edge even with the end of the toe.

Although warm foot soaks can relieve inflammation and soften the nail for easier trimming, home remedies should not be continued if pain or inflammation (swelling, redness, tenderness, local heat, or discharge) persist.

Your doctor may offer conservative medical treatment. Warm soapy soaks might be continued. An antibiotic can be prescribed for infection. Pushing small bits of cotton moistened with petroleum jelly under the corners of the nail will elevate it and prevent further irritation of the surrounding skin. Surgery (usually performed under local anesthesia in the doctor's or podiatrist's office) involves removal of the nail margin and sometimes a portion of the nail bed where the nail is formed. Recovery should occur rapidly but may require the use of a cutout shoe or open sandal, as well as dressing changes with an antibiotic solution or ointment and perhaps even further soaking. Very occasionally more extensive surgery is needed, which can be performed as a hospital outpatient. If a nail falls off because of injury or has to be removed surgically, another will grow in its place if the nail bed is not injured. Depending on one's age, this can take six to nine months.

Corns and Calluses

Corns and calluses are skin thickenings over pressure points. Calluses are often found on the soles, whereas corns commonly occur on the toes. "Hard" corns develop at pressure points, such as over the joint of a hammertoe; "soft" corns develop on opposing toe surfaces as a result of local heat and moisture. Corns and calluses are painful, particularly when there is a deep core (seed) in the center. This "seed" can be very firm and must be removed for relief of pain.

Over-the-counter medicines should not be used to dissolve corns because these frequently contain irritating acids. Never trim your corns or calluses with a sharp object such as a razor blade or scissors. Healthy skin can easily be damaged and infection can occur.

Corns and calluses are treated by (1) wearing proper shoes that do not cause pressure, (2) soaking the feet in warm (not hot) soapy water), (3) using appropriate cushions or pads, (4) sanding calluses with a fine emery board or a pumice stone, and (5) professional trimming. When conservative treatment fails, surgery is available. Surgery usually involves removing an underlying bony excrescence or changing the position of a small toe bone.

Plantar Warts

A plantar wart is a virus-induced skin growth on the sole of the foot. It is characterized by a central circular crater containing small black dots. These spots are actually blood clots in the small blood vessels that come to the surface of the skin. A plantar wart can be painful. It usually has a life cycle that depends on the infecting virus. This may be as long as one to two years.

There are numerous folk remedies for warts, most of which depend on strong suggestibility on the part of the patient. Even Tom Sawyer had a suggestion that involved backing up to a river stump, placing the wart under water, and reciting, "Barleycorn, barleycorn, Injun-meal shorts, skunk-water, skunk-water, swallow these warts!" However, plantar warts do not often respond to home remedies. Sequential applications of acids and pads by your doctor may soften the wart and relieve some of the pain. Large (mosaic) warts can be treated by soaking in a diluted solution of formalin. Only the wart-bearing tissue is immersed for 5 to 15 minutes each night. The toes must be protected with petroleum jelly. Laser (**L**ight **A**mplification by **S**timulated **E**mission of **R**adiation) and ultrasound (mechanical waves converted to deep heat) destruction or surgical excision are available for highly recalcitrant warts.

Athlete's Foot

. *Athlete's foot* (tinea pedis) is a fungal infection and, like plantar warts, is easily transmittable through shower or locker room contamination. In either of these conditions, it is wise to avoid contact with the eyes, other parts of the body, or other persons, and by observing hygienic measures to minimize spread of the infection.

Athlete's foot leads to painful itching and scaling, with redness and blistering. Frequent washing and drying of the feet, regular changes of hosiery, and the use of an antifungal cream and powder may be all that is necessary for successful treatment. If not, a doctor (usually a dermatologist) should be consulted.

Heel Pain

Most cases of heel pain are due to a chronic inflammation of the *plantar fascia,* a thick ligament that stretches from the heel to the forefoot. This can be a particular problem in people with high arches in whom the fascia tends to be tight, just as a bowstring is tight when the bow is bent. An x-ray may or may not show a bony spur. Treatment involves the use of an appropriate pad, which can be fashioned from soft felt or foam rubber (scraps can be obtained at small cost from an upholsterer's shop, or a kitchen sponge can be used). Special heel cups made of either plastic or soft rubber are designed to compact the heel pad and distribute weight over the entire supporting surface of the heel, thus avoiding point pressure. An injection of cortisone and local anesthetic (Novocain or

Xylocaine) into the area of inflammation is sometimes neces-sary. This may be augmented with oral anti-inflammatory medication. Surgery (removal of a spur or thickened plantar fascia) is seldom indicated.

Arch Pain

As mentioned previously, a flat foot, known to your doctor as *pes planus* (foot flat), has a dropped long arch. Most flat feet are of the flexible or functional type. There seems to be a hered-itary disposition toward flatfoot. This is expressed in looseness of the foot ligaments or abnormalities in the shape of the bones of the feet. Not all flat feet are painful. Flatfooted people seldom suffer from plantar fasciitis because their plantar fascia is not tight enough to strain. They may even be better off than are those who have high arched feet because they can absorb walking shocks over a larger surface. You can check your own arches by making footprints with your damp feet on a piece of newspaper. Normal feet leave a mark approximately one inch wide at the middle of the foot. Flat feet will leave a mark the entire width of your foot and high arches will leave a thin mark or none at all.

Treatment of flat feet is usually through prescription shoes, appropriate arch supports, and exercise. Operations are avail-able but seldom indicated.

A depressed short or metatarsal arch can cause abnormal pressure on the ball of the foot. The depressed arch can often be elevated by metatarsal pads that fit inside the shoe or by metatarsal bars that are attached to the sole of the shoe. Special shoes, referred to as *heel-negative* (the heel is lower than normal) are designed to relieve weight bearing in the forefoot.

Surgery may be necessary if pain persists. This entails either removing that part of the metatarsal head that is causing pressure on weight bearing or cutting the metatarsal bone near the head and allowing it to heal with the metatarsal head ele-vated, thus relieving a pressure point in the sole.

Hammertoes

A muscle imbalance that causes the ends of the smaller toes to bend down, aggravated by tight-fitting shoes, may cause a hammer deformity of the inside joint of a toe. This results in a painful callus at the tip of the toe and a painful corn where it is angulated upward and presses on the shoe. This condition is called a hammertoe because the deformity looks like one of the hammers that strike the strings in a piano. It is distinguished from a "mallet toe" in which the bent toe joint is the one near the tip. Proper treatment for hammertoe is surgical, consisting of the removal of bone and lengthening of tendons. This can usually be performed on an outpatient basis under local anesthesia. Recovery is within three to four weeks. When surgery cannot be performed for whatever reason, the patient can use an open shoe or have a special shoe constructed to conform to the shape of the foot. This is called a "space boot," and although it is not particularly attractive, it is very comfortable. Whereas the standard shoe expects the foot to conform to its shape, "space boots" are designed to fit only one pair of feet. A cast of the foot is taken, and the shoe fashioned on a last made from the cast. "Space boots" are usually oxfords. They are fabricated with very supple leathers (often deerskin uppers) and have cushioned soles and a supporting insert made of light plastic foam. They close on the side by laces or velcro and are very light and easy to wear.

SIX RULES TO KEEP YOU ON YOUR FEET

1. Bathe your feet at least once a day for ten minutes in warm water and follow with a brisk cold cream massage.

2. Use alternating foot baths of warm and cold water, starting and ending in the warm water, spending two minutes in the warm and then one minute in the cold for a period of eleven minutes.

3. Rest your feet whenever you can. When sitting, cross your legs and rest your feet on their outside borders. When possible, lie down and elevate your feet higher than the rest of your body.

4. Exercise your feet frequently by wiggling the toes vigorously, moving your ankle and foot up and down, in and out. Try to pick up a pencil, clothespin, or marbles with the toes, or attempt to crumple a small piece of light paper or a washrag.

5. Wear proper foot wear. Be sure your shoes are well fitted and wide and long enough for comfort.

6. Pare your toenails properly, in a straight line and relatively long. Sand any calluses with a pumice stone during the bath or a fine emery board when dry.

Morton's Neuroma

The term *Morton's neuroma* (plantar neuroma), named for a military surgeon during the Civil War who founded the Philadelphia Orthopaedic Hospital and in 1887 performed one of the first appendectomies, after seeing his son and brother die of untreated appendicitis (he himself died of cholera in Philadelphia), is a misnomer. A neuroma is a tumor of nerve. Morton's neuroma is a localized swelling of a nerve going to the toes that is caused by pressure between the metatarsal heads. Symptoms include pain into several toes (usually the third and fourth) as well as numbness due to constant pressure on the nerve. A person with a Morton's neuroma often feels as if he or she has a small pebble in the shoe.

Plantar neuroma sometimes responds to local anti-inflammatory drugs and a change to a wider shoe. The condition is found most frequently in women who wear high heels. Help may sometimes be obtained simply by lowering the heel height. A local injection of steroid into the area of swelling often provides relief. Surgical excision of the neuroma can be performed as an outpatient under local anesthesia. The enlarged portion of the nerve is removed, which results in some permanent numbness in the area of its supply. However, this is a small price to pay for relief from an annoying, persistently painful foot condition.

Bunions

A bunion, or *hallux valgus* (great toe—bent out), is a deformity of the large toe. It is more common in women than in men and tends to run in families. Bunions are *de rigeur* for dancers, an adaptation to the pointed shoes into which they force their feet. An unsightly bump develops at the base of the big toe, where the joint angles inward. Because bunions increase the width of the forefoot, the bony area of the bunion is irritated where the shoe presses against it. An inflamed bursa forms beneath the skin at this point. A bunion can become so deformed that it forces the second toe into an overlapping hammertoe position. It should be obvious that cramming the foot into a narrow pointed toe box with a high heel will aggravate a bunion, and indeed it does. People who have arthritis, particularly of the rheumatoid type, or flatfoot are more prone to develop bunions.

Self-care of bunions includes wearing shoes wide enough to accommodate the bunion deformity and the use of a soft toe support or "bunion post." Warm foot soaks are also helpful in decreasing inflammation, an analgesic such as aspirin may relieve pain, and ultrasound or whirlpool baths can be helpful. However, the only definitive care for a bunion is surgical. An operation called a bunionectomy is performed in a hospital setting. Although not all bunions require surgical correction, an operation may be necessary when there is severe deformity and pain and increased difficulty in fitting shoes. Although this can be done under local anesthesia, it may require a spinal or general anesthetic. Surgery involves removing the bunion bump and realigning the great toe. This may necessitate correcting the deformity by cutting the bone and resetting it in the corrected position. Soft tissue reconstruction of ligaments that have been stretched out of shape may also be necessary.

Resecting bone at the bunion joint is another surgical alternative that removes a focus of arthritic irritation. Yet another option is to replace the involved joint with a prosthetic implant that acts as a joint filler, usually the bio-inert plastic Silastic, or metal titanium. This keeps the bones separated and properly aligned, maintaining the length of the toe but still allows for toe flexibility. Such surgery can be performed as an outpatient but often requires a day in the hospital because some pain and swelling occurs after the operation. The foot is kept elevated and may be in a bulky pressure dressing or cast. Occasionally a pin is used to maintain the position of the realigned bones. This is removed two to three weeks after surgery. Rehabilitation after bunion surgery is somewhat prolonged. Although the patient can often walk immediately in a cast and after cast removal in a special shoe, it may take as long as three months for healing to be complete and standing and walking in a normal fashion to be possible.

A cousin to the bunion is a bunionette (or "tailor's bunion," so called because tailors used to sit cross-legged on the floor, which irritated the outer margins of their feet), an outer angulation at the base of the fifth toe that produces a painful bump. This can also be treated with a shoe of proper width, but surgical removal of the bony prominence is a simple procedure that can be performed on an outpatient basis, does not require a cast, and is safe and usually effective.

Another member of the bunion family is a condition called *hallux rigidus*—rigidity of the great toe. This is characterized by swelling, pain, and sometimes redness at the base of the toe, but there is no angulation or bump as in a bunion. Hallux rigidus is due to arthritis at the base of the toe, which may result from either a single injury or repeated stress. The condition sometimes responds to oral anti-inflammatory medication and a steroid injection. Wearing a shoe that has a rigid sole or a special splint may prevent excess motion at this joint, decreasing pain. Surgery for hallux rigidus involves removal of one surface of the joint, and resurfacing with a prosthetic implant is sometimes performed.

The Diabetic Foot

Even mild diabetes may eventually cause damage to nerves and blood vessels, which can lead to decreased sensation and circulation in the feet. Pressure sores, ulcers, and infection result. Prevention is possible through close surveillance of the feet with daily inspection and immediate treatment of any scratches, abrasions, or pressure areas. Good foot hygiene is mandatory. The feet should be washed in warm (not hot) soapy water, dried thoroughly, and powdered with a mild talcum powder. A nonirritating moisturizing cream or lotion should be used daily to maintain skin tone and suppleness. Nails must be given proper care (see section on nail care), and shoes should be light and comfortable. Extremes of temperature as well as strong chemicals such as those often found in corn removers should be avoided. Needless to say, the diabetes should be kept under control with proper diet and oral medications or insulin. In the case of advanced damage to the feet, which may include damage to the bones and joints as well as the skin, hospitalization with bed rest, elevation of the feet, and intravenous administration of antibiotics becomes necessary. Casting of the damaged foot as well as surgery to remove infected bone and in some cases amputation may be indicated.

We often tend to forget our feet until, through pain and disability, they remind us of how important they are to our well-being. By developing an awareness of the importance of foot care and following some simple procedures, such as wearing proper shoes, employing daily foot hygiene, trimming nails properly, seeking help from your doctor when self-care of a foot problem is inadequate, your feet will remain your friends.

What the feet are to the legs, the hands are to the arms. Let's take a look.

QUESTIONS AND ANSWERS ABOUT THE FEET

Q: My little girl takes ballet lessons. When is it safe to let her go "on point?"

A: This gives rise to much controversy. Some ballet teachers refuse to put a student on her toes until a certain age. Others are more flexible, putting a child "on point" based on her individual talent. The age that is most frequently given is 12 years. This, however, depends on having significant training, and it may be that with such training a child considerably younger is ready to go on her toes. Some children should never go on their toes, whereas others seem to be born with the ability to perform "on point." In the final analysis, trust in the ballet instructor's judgment is probably the most important variable in deciding when a student should go "on point."

Q: Can corns predict the weather?

A: Some say they do. Any change in atmospheric pressure will cause a change of pressure in a bursal sac near a corn (also in the closed synovial lined spaces of joints). Pain lets you know that there will be a change in the weather.

Q: What causes a blister on the foot?

A: Friction between the shoe and the skin causes a blister. A blister is actually a protective fluid-filled pad that is the body's defense against the friction caused by the foot moving within the shoe. You can prevent blisters by having shoes that fit well. Once a blister is formed, it should be cleansed with an antiseptic solution such as Betadine, and punctured with a sterile sharp instrument (a needle sterilized with a match flame will do). The top part of the blister should be left in place, an antibiotic cream (e.g., Bacitracin) applied, and the blister covered with a sterile bandage. Never minimize the potential harm a blister can do. In the 1979 Grand Prix Master's Tennis Tournament, Jimmy Connors was forced to default by a painful blister on his foot, giving up his chance to win the $100,000 first prize!

Q: What is a "pump bump?"

A: A "pump bump" is an irritation of the tissue at the back of the heel, such as that caused by a firm counter in a pump shoe. An inflamed bursal sac may result from the shoe rubbing against the bump, or there may be a reactive overgrowth of bone. Treatment consists of softening the heel counter, placing a heel pad in the shoe to lift the foot up and away from the irritating counteredge, and using warm moist applications. Extreme bony growth may need to be removed surgically.

Q: Are women particularly vulnerable to foot strain during pregnancy?

A: Yes, for two reasons. In the first place, they place excessive weight on their feet. Second, there is an excess of the female hormone relaxin, which creates ligamentous laxity. This is necessary so that the pelvis can stretch to allow passage of the baby during birth. However, at the same time the pelvic ligaments are relaxing, ligaments elsewhere in the body are also weakened, including those of the foot. Incidentally, women have more rearfoot motion due to increased pronation (flattening) as well as a normal greater laxity of their ligaments, which can lead to considerable foot strain.

Q: What is reflexology? Does it work?

A: Reflexology is the practice of foot massage to improve health in other parts of the body. This theory holds that there are points on the foot that relate to the organs of the body. Like hypnosis, reflexology seems to give the best results in people who are suggestible.

Q: Are overlapping toes a serious problem?

A: Approximately 25 percent of babies have a toe that lies either over or under its neighbor. This is most common when the fifth toe overlaps the fourth. This is not a serious condition and can be remedied by taping the toe into the corrected position and stretching it frequently. If neglected and bothersome, overlapping toes can be corrected surgically.

13

The Hand

Hand, N. A singular instrument worn at the end of the human arm
and commonly thrust into somebody's pocket.

Ambrose Bierce
The Devil's Dictionary

We often take our hands for granted, yet they are a most
remarkable and invaluable part of our anatomy. Hands can
sometimes perform unbelievable feats of dexterity. More of the
brain is committed to movements of the hand than any other
motor task. Because our hands are used so often, they are frequently at risk for injury. Falls can produce sprains, strains, and
fractures of the wrist or fingers. Cuts and crushing injuries can
occur. The hand can be the site of any kind of trauma or disease.
Statistically the index (pointer) finger of the nondominant hand
is the digit most frequently injured in industrial or household
accidents.

There are 27 bones in the hand and wrist (Figure 13-1).
Those of the hand proper are labeled with the oxymoron *short-
long bones.* The eight wrist bones, or *carpals,* articulate so as to
provide smooth motion at the wrist, between the long bones of
the forearm (the radius and the ulna) and the metacarpal bones
of the palm, one for each finger. Have you ever noticed that
Mickey Mouse and the other Disney animal characters only have
four fingers? This saves hundreds of thousands of man hours of
work during the illustration of an animated movie. The thumb
has two additional bones (phalanges), and the other four fingers
each have three (Figure 13-2). The term *phalanges* is from the
Greek for a band of soldiers drawn up for battle. Not an inap-

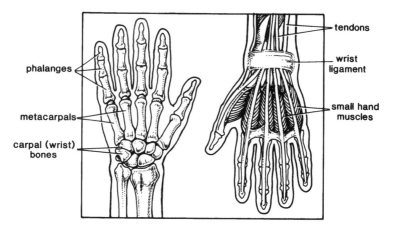

FIGURE 13-1 Anatomy of the Hand

propriate description considering the function some hands are put to. Incidentally, there is no agreement on nomenclature for the hand. Is the thumb the first finger? Do we have five fingers or only four? Which, then, is the forefinger? Although most of the separate states have adopted standard systems of naming the digits, 10 different systems are in use. Nonetheless, our medical and legal systems seem to muddle through.

The *equiangular spiral* (a logarithmic curve), so perfectly illustrated in the shell of the chambered nautilus and the shape of the egg, allows for the almost limitless ability of the hand to grasp. This curve is determined by interarticular ratios of the small bones of the hand, which closely follow a Fibonacci sequence (0, 1, 1, 2, 3, 5, 8, 13 . . .). This ratio (1:1.618) is also seen in the golden rectangle of classical Greek architecture. Thus has nature fitted man with a superb instrument to serve such exquisite diversity of function and expression.

FIGURE 13-2 Normal Finger Anatomy

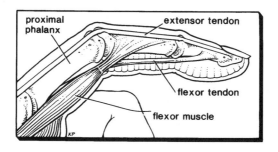

The hand holds a group of small so-called *intrinsic muscles.* Long muscles originating at the elbow and ending in thin tendons both extend the fingers or flex them into a fist. In addition to keenly tuned motor function permitting very fine movement with great strength, the hand is provided with an unusual array of sensory nerve endings that detect temperature, pressure, position, and pain. Mobility in the joints of the hand is assured by a variety of ligaments and other fibrous structures that align and stabilize the bones.

The human hand is unique in that the thumb can be brought to each finger; *opposition* has played an integral part in human development. It is our ability to oppose our thumbs that grants us the skill to grasp tools and perform other functional tasks with our hands, distinguishing us from our primate cousins, the large apes. Proper function of the hand requires the ability to grasp and release the grip. Function is broadly categorized into power grasp (prehension), large cylindrical and small cylindrical holding, hooking, fine fingertip opposition, and bringing all the fingertips together in the form of a chuck. These skills enable the human hand to perform its many tasks.

What is most remarkable is that the hand possesses two distinct grips. For instance, two balls can be separately held by different parts of a single hand. A bottle can be held and its cap unscrewed by the same hand. This dexterity adds dimensions to the operations of the human hand far beyond those of simpler functions. Even the appellation *surgeon* is derived from the Greek *cheir* (hand) plus *ergon* (work).

The injured hand may be seen and treated by an orthopaedic surgeon. Complicated wounds may require a specialist in hand surgery. Rehabilitation is often provided by a physical or occupational therapist. An injury to the hand, like any other injury, will require evaluation through a history and physical examination, an x-ray, and perhaps special tests such as a CT scan or MRI.

SOME COMMON CONDITIONS AND INJURIES OF THE HAND AND WRIST

1. *Fingertip crush.* Such an injury can fracture the small end bone (distal phalanx) in the fingertip. There is often soft tissue crushing as well as severe damage to the nail. The finger

is cleaned and dead tissue carefully removed. The nail is usually left in place. A padded splint is applied. When there is no bony or serious soft tissue injury but only a blood clot deep to the nail, the blood can be drained through a hole drilled in the nail. A splint may or may not be indicated.

2. *Fingertip loss.* A fingertip that has been cut by a sharp instrument may sometimes be sewn back. When larger portions of a finger have been amputated, the amputated part should be wrapped in a cloth moistened with salt water, placed in ice, and taken to the emergency room with the patient as soon as possible. Often such a finger can be saved and sewn back. This involves special microsurgical techniques by which the small blood vessels to the finger are reapproximated with fine stitches. A small skin graft can be applied if only the skin at the fingertip has been lost or, in many instances, nonadherent dressings over a period of two to three weeks will allow new skin to cover the open wound.

3. *Lacerations.* Minor lacerations that involve only the skin should be cleaned and closed with fine sutures or tapes. These usually heal within a week or so. Deeper lacerations may cut nerves, blood vessels, or tendons. Severed tendons can be stitched. Those tendons that extend (straighten) the fingers are more easily repaired. Those that flex (bend) the fingers are more difficult because scar tissue may bind the tendon in its tunnel. For this type of problem, the surgeon sometimes elects to perform a tendon graft, replacing the old tendon with a new one. Tendon surgery is accompanied by brief splinting followed by active motion of the tendon augmented by physical therapy to prevent scarring by maintaining movement.

4. *Nerve compression syndromes.* Either the median or ulnar nerve entering the hand may be compressed, causing weakness and numbness. The most common nerve compression syndrome in the hand is *carpal tunnel syndrome,* which results from pressure on the median nerve as it enters the hand deep to the palmar surface of the wrist. In order to gain access to the fingers, the nerve must pass underneath a bridge of thick fibrous tissue called the *transverse volar carpal ligament,* which arches between several carpal (wrist) bones, forming the roof of a tunnel called the carpal tunnel. Tendons also pass through the

tunnel, which makes the anatomy rather tight, and anything pressing into or causing swelling in the tunnel can squeeze the nerve at the wrist. Some common causes of such pressure are:

❏ wear and tear due to repetitive movements, which produces thickening of the soft tissues in the tunnel;
❏ dislocation or fracture at the wrist, which causes bone to protrude into the tunnel;
❏ fluid retention, which generates swelling in the tunnel (this often occurs during pregnancy and subsides after delivery);
❏ arthritis of the wrist; and
❏ tumors.

Carpal tunnel syndrome is a frequent cause of work-related disability. The "repetitive strain syndrome" seen in typists or computer technicians is well known. Workers who use tools should try to keep their wrists positioned at neutral, avoiding unusual strain by using a firm grip at all times. Frequent rest periods, minimizing repetitive tasks, support of the forearm while typing or using a computer, reducing force and speed in wrist movement, and conditioning exercises all help carpal tunnel syndrome. The syndrome is characterized by pain in the wrist with numbness of the thumb, index, and middle fingers. Symptoms often are worse at night.

Examination includes physical tests such as gently tapping over the nerve (Tinel's sign), which causes a mild electrical shocklike feeling in the involved fingers, and positioning the wrist in a flexed (bent down) position (Phalen's sign), which quickly aggravates the symptoms. X-rays rule out contributing bony conditions, and electrical tests may be ordered. These may include a nerve conduction velocity test, which measures the speed of electrical conduction along the nerve—it is reduced in carpal tunnel syndrome, and the electromyogram, which reveals abnormalities in muscles—it is positive in the base of the thumb muscles involved in carpal tunnel syndrome. Thermography, the measurement of heat radiating from the hand, is also useful in the diagnosis of this condition.

The treatment of carpal tunnel syndrome includes putting the hand at rest with a splint, anti-inflammatory medication, occasionally diuretics or vitamin B6, and often the injection of a steroid drug directly into the carpal tunnel in an attempt to decrease swelling and inflammation in the tunnel itself.

Many cases of carpal tunnel syndrome will respond to these conservative measures. Those that do not require a carpal tunnel release. This is a relatively simple operation, usually performed under local anesthesia, either directly or through an endoscope. The median nerve is identified and protected as the transverse volar carpal ligament is transected, easing pressure on the nerve.

Postoperative recovery involves using a splint for approximately one week, elevation of the arm to prevent swelling, and rehabilitation exercises to improve strength in the hand.

5. *Sprains.* Sprains of the wrist are common and should be treated vigorously because undertreatment can result in chronic instability and/or disability of the wrist. X-rays may reveal separation of one or several wrist bones. This must be corrected by manipulation. A plaster cast often will hold the corrected position until healing is complete, but an operation with pin fixation is sometimes necessary.

A sprain can occur in any finger joint. A common injury is a tear of one of the collateral (side) ligaments of the thumb. These ligaments run along the base of the thumb, stabilizing it as it moves. Such sprains are often successfully treated by immobilization in a splint or cast, but surgical repair may be necessary if a ligament is severely torn.

"Gamekeeper's thumb" is an injury (often a tear) of the ulnar (inside) collateral ligament of the thumb. Gamekeepers used to kill animals such as rabbits by snapping their necks between their thumb and index finger, stretching and injuring this ligament, hence the eponym. Today it is an athletic injury that occurs mostly in skiing, from improper use of a ski pole, or in football, from blocking with the hands or falling on the thumb.

6. *Hand and wrist fractures.* Direct blows or crushing injuries can cause fractures of any of the hand bones. Fractures of the phalanges are usually treated with manipulation and reduction and held in functional splints. Proper realignment is vital, particularly in rotation, and may require an operation with open reduction and pins or a small plate and screws to maintain position.

Mallet finger is caused by an avulsion of the extensor tendon with or without a small chip of bone, causing the fingertip to drop.

This frequently happens when one attempts to pull sheets tight while making a bed. Such activity involves strong bending of the fingertips and when the finger is suddenly released the injury can occur. Treatment is by splinting the fingertip straight for at least six weeks. Operative correction occasionally is necessary.

The metacarpal bones may be broken in their shaft portion. If they are severe, these fractures are treated with casts or surgery. A common fracture of the metacarpal occurs at its neck, with angulation of the metacarpal head into the palm. This is called a boxer's fracture, as it is seen frequently when someone strikes a hard surface (such as a face or a wall) with a clenched fist, thus breaking the bone at the knuckle. Almost all boxer's fractures are treated by closed reduction and casting for three to six weeks.

Although any of the carpal bones can be broken, and often are, the most frequently injured and one of the most serious fractures to these bones is that of the carpal navicular bone. The break usually results from a fall on the flexed wrist. Fractures of the scaphoid (navicular), so called because it has the appearance of a skiff or boat: Greek = *scaphos* or Latin = navicular (hence the word *Navy*), can be serious because this bone has a tenuous blood supply which, if interrupted, can lead to necrosis—death—of a portion of the bone. Scaphoid fractures are frequently not initially apparent, which is why every serious wrist injury should be splinted and re-x-rayed 7 to 10 days later, to see if a fracture line appears. Treatment of scaphoid fractures involves immobilization with a cast for anywhere up to six months. If the fracture does not heal, surgery with screw fixation and/or bone grafting may be necessary. Local electrical stimulation also has been used to treat nonunion of these fractures.

A jammed finger due to a direct blow, such as that incurred when trying to field a baseball, can cause considerable injury, particularly to the joint between the first and second phalanx. The ends of the phalanx can be chipped or broken. A chip often indicates that a ligament has pulled off. Reduction and splinting with early range of motion exercises is usually recommended.

A hard fall directly on the thumb can tear the ligaments at its base, accompanied by a fracture of the articular surface at the thumb carpal-metacarpal joint. This is called a Bennett's fracture, and although closed reduction with casting is usually successful, it is often necessary to hold the fracture with a pin placed under x-ray control through the skin and across the fracture site.

As function of the thumb is one of the things that distinguishes us from the ape, it is vital that this fracture be properly reduced so that it can heal in the best possible anatomic position.

A break of the end of the two forearm bones at the wrist is a Colles' fracture, named after the nineteenth century Irish surgeon who first described it. Clean breaks can often be reduced closed and held in a long or short arm plaster cast for six weeks followed by a vigorous exercise program to regain motion. Sometimes the fracture is *comminuted* (many pieces) or otherwise unstable, and had best be held by pins held by an external fixator apparatus. Open reduction with metallic fixation using plates and screws or pins occasionally is necessary to hold the bone fragments together until union occurs.

The arm should be elevated to decrease swelling after reduction of a Colles' fracture. The fingers must be moved to maintain circulation and motion. The shoulder also should be exercised so that it does not become stiff. Any unusual finger swelling, pain, discoloration (paleness or blueness) or tingling (these are the four P's—**P**uffiness, **P**ain, **P**allor, and **P**aresthesia [pins and needles feeling]) should be reported immediately to your doctor because they are indications that the cast is too tight and may require splitting for relief.

These are only some of the many orthopaedic problems that can occur in the hand and wrist. Of course, the best medicine is prevention, and you should observe safety precautions at home and at work to avoid harm. In the case of injuries, even minor ones, prompt treatment will prevent more serious damage and subsequent disability. Cooperating with a supervised rehabilitation program after treatment can help restore the most function to the hand in the shortest possible time.

Now let's take up some loose ends to make our *All About Bone* review complete.

QUESTIONS AND ANSWERS ABOUT THE HAND

> *Q:* What should I remember when giving first aid for a hand injury?
>
> *A:* The important things to remember are:
>
> > ❏ do not attempt to cleanse the wound if it appears at all serious; simply apply pressure over a sterile or clean pad to control bleeding;

❑ place a roll of bandage or other material into the victim's palm and curve his fingers around it;

❑ separate the fingers by gauze or cloth dressing material and cover the entire hand with a clean towel or cloth or an unused plastic bag;

❑ keep the hand elevated above the level of the heart during transportation to receive medical care in order to further reduce swelling. Only after insect stings or snake bite should the hand be kept hanging down after injury. If a finger has been cut off and is salvageable, wrap it in gauze soaked in salt water and transport it on ice to the emergency room.

Q: What are some simple ways to splint fractures of the hand for transportation to an emergency room?

A: A fractured hand can be easily splinted in a pillow or supported on a tightly folded newspaper. A wooden tongue blade may be used to splint a broken finger. If no splinting material is available, you can splint a broken finger simply by bandaging it to an adjacent uninjured digit.

Q: Where do the most serious hand injuries occur?

A: The most serious hand injuries undoubtedly occur in industrial or agricultural accidents. Hands crushed in punch presses or mangled in corn pickers present serious reconstructive challenges to specialists in hand surgery.

Q: Are there orthopaedic techniques for restoring function to severely congenitally deformed hands or those that have been badly injured?

A: Yes. Operations are available for fusing unstable joints, transferring tendons to provide increased range of motion, releasing contractures, and grafting skin to cover wounds. Where amputation is necessary, prostheses are not only cosmetically acceptable but can be motivated electrically or through muscle connections higher up in the arm.

Q: What is Dupuytren's contracture? What is de Quervain's disease?

A: Dupuytren's contracture was named after a famous nineteenth century French surgeon, Guillaime Dupuytren. It is chronic scarring of the fascia of the palm, leading to painless bending of the fingers into the palm. Its cause is uncertain and it chiefly affects adult men, often of Irish or Scottish ancestry. This was the condition for which President Ronald Reagan was operated on during his last few weeks in office. Reagan is a descendant of Irish immigrants.

De Quervain was yet another French surgeon who first described tendinitis of the wrist affecting the tendons connecting the thumb to the muscles of the forearm, hence the eponym.

Q: Can "cracking" the knuckles cause joint damage or arthritis?

A: In an otherwise healthy hand, "cracking" the knuckles is not hazardous and does not cause arthritis. Some scientists think that the "cracking" or "snapping" sound is caused by a ligament, tendon, or joint capsule sliding over a bony protuberance. Others trace the popping to the bursting of gas bubbles that are released when the joint is stretched, reducing pressure on its contained synovial fluid. The gas is only slowly resorbed, so you cannot crack your knuckles again for 15 minutes or so. Many joints other than those in the hand (e.g., toes, knees, hips, shoulders, and neck) can be "cracked" in this fashion. Although the sound may be annoying, or even frightening, if it is unaccompanied by pain, numbness, or muscle spasms, the practice is not dangerous. There is no treatment except the use of ear plugs.

14

Congenital Diseases of Bone

Is this the poultice for my aching bones?

William Shakespeare
Romeo and Juliet

A *hereditary* disease is one that is genetically determined, while a *congenital* disease is simply one that is present at birth. Some congenital bone diseases are hereditary, but many others are caused by an abnormality that occurs during pregnancy.

Either partial or total absence of certain bones can occur. This is most frequent in the bones of the forearm and that of the thigh. Congenital *pseudarthrosis* (false joint) of the shin bone (tibia) is also seen. Treatment of these conditions consists of surgical procedures to obtain union, integrity, and proper length of the bone using special fixation equipment and bone grafting. Such conditions are often difficult to treat and some eventually require limb amputation.

Osteogenesis imperfecta, also called *fragilitas ossium,* is just that—fragile bones. This familial disease is characterized by bones that are easily broken, leading to short stature and skeletal deformity. The French artist Toulouse-Lautrec may have had osteogenesis imperfecta.

Widespread abnormalities of the growth centers is hereditary. One example is a type of stunted growth called *achondroplastic dwarfism.* People with this disease have short extremities and a large head and trunk. They are otherwise well and active. These are the "dwarfs" who were at one time frequently seen in carnivals and circuses. Inbreeding of this condition in dogs produces the sausage-bodied, short-legged Dachshund.

Another hereditary bony disorder is Marfan's syndrome, an abnormality of the elastic and collagen tissue. The extremities are long, thin, and spider-like. Abraham Lincoln was reputed to suffer from this problem.

Club feet and congenital hip dislocation are intrauterine abnormalities. These conditions are probably due to mechanical factors acting on the embryo while carried in the uterus. Club feet are more prevalent in boys, whereas congenital hip dislocation is seen more frequently in girls. (Congenital hip dislocation also is a frequent problem in highly inbred pedigreed dogs such as the dalmatian, greyhound, or Irish setter.) Manipulation and corrective bracing or casting may be used initially in both conditions, in the club foot to mold and maintain the foot in its proper position and in the dislocated hip to relocate and hold the hip bone in place until growth has formed an adequate hip socket. However, more severe cases of club foot or dislocated hip, or those seen late, require surgical correction.

BONE TUMOR

A tumor is called a *neoplasm* (*neo:* new, *plasm:* anything formed). Tumors in bone are either primary (that is, arising first in bone) or metastatic (secondary) from malignancies elsewhere in the body. Metastatic tumors are by far the most common neoplasms found in bone. They are all malignant. The usual sources of metastatic tumor to bone are cancers of the lung, prostate, breast, kidney, and thyroid.

Primary bone tumors arise from skeletal tissues themselves (bone, cartilage, fibrous tissue). They may either be malignant or benign, and they are characterized by the skeletal tissue element from which they originate. For example, bone tissue can give rise to a malignant osteosarcoma (the tumor that Senator Edward Kennedy's son had) or benign osteoma, cartilage can form a malignant chondrosarcoma or a benign chondroma, and fibrous tissue can produce a malignant fibrosarcoma or a benign fibroma. The suffix *sarcoma* derives from the Greek *sarc* (fleshy) plus *oma* (tumor). *Osteo,* of course, refers to bone, *chondro* to cartilage, and *fibro* to fibrous tissue. Finally, tumors also occur from bone marrow, including the malignant myeloma and the benign eosinophilic granuloma. Incidentally, malignant myeloma is the most common primary malignancy of bone.

The signs and symptoms of bone tumor are localized swelling, redness, and pain. A pathologic fracture can occur because bone is often weakened by a tumor. Diagnosis is usually made by x-ray or other imaging and confirmed by biopsy. Tumors occasionally can be detected by examination of blood or other body fluids because certain primary or secondary tumors cause chemical abnormalities, such as an elevation in the blood enzyme alkaline phosphatase in osteosarcoma or the presence of the abnormal Bence-Jones protein in the urine in multiple myeloma.

Benign bone tumors usually require no more than local resection and bone grafting. Malignant tumors can sometimes be treated by wide local resection with limb salvage, which often requires prosthetic replacement and/or bone grafting. Amputation may be necessary if invasion of the tumor is advanced.

Surgical treatment is usually augmented with radiation or chemotherapy. The treatment of metastatic bone tumors aims to prevent fracture and repair local damage to the bone.

TOTAL JOINT REPLACEMENT

The earliest documented total joint replacement was performed by Theophilus Gluck, a German surgeon who in 1891 replaced a diseased hip with an ivory ball and socket, which he screwed into place. The artificial hip dislocated almost immediately on weight bearing. The late Sir John Charnley, a contemporary English orthopaedist, pioneered in the development of materials and techniques for total joint replacement. In this procedure, an arthritic or damaged joint is replaced with a prosthetic or artificial one. More than one-quarter of a million joints are replaced annually worldwide. In the United States alone approximately 100,000 total knee replacements are performed each year. Total joint replacement most commonly involves the hip or the knee because these joints are most frequently affected by degenerative and rheumatoid arthritis. However, devices have been developed for replacement of the shoulder, fingers, ankle, wrist, and elbow, as well as for as partial replacement of joints about the foot.

The technique of total joint replacement involves implanting a device that resurfaces and replaces the degenerated articular surfaces of the joint. Most total joints are composed of a hard plastic portion made of high density polyethylene matched with a metallic component, usually an alloy of cobalt, chrome, and titanium or stainless steel. These parts are cemented into the joint after it is prepared to receive them. Joint replacements that do not require cement but rely on bony ingrowth into a specially treated metal surface incorporating metal beads or fibers have been developed and are increasingly used, particularly in younger patients.

The goal of joint replacement is to correct the disability that results from pain, malalignment of the joint, and loss of motion. The operation can be performed in adults with degenerative arthritis and in adults and children with rheumatoid arthritis. Many patients have had four or five of their joints replaced. Advanced age is no contraindication to surgery, and recovery following a joint replacement is usually rapid. In the case of a total hip or knee replacement, the average patient is encouraged to stand and walk within a few days after surgery. Hospitalization normally is followed by a home exercise program that continues for several months. A cane or crutches may be necessary to protect the joint during rehabilitation.

A total knee or hip replacement operation can take several hours and may require a blood transfusion. Many patients elect to donate their own blood before entering the hospital so that it is available for the transfusion if necessary. Operative risks include blood clots and pneumonia. A most dangerous complication after operation is infection. This may be superficial or deep and can occur during the hospital stay or even several years afterward. Superficial infections can be treated locally but deep infections may require further surgery for drainage or even removal of the prosthesis. Because spread of infection from another part of the body can occur, people who have total joint replacements are given antibiotics before dental work (including cleaning the teeth) or other types of surgery. Late complications include loosening of the prosthesis, which may require replacement; dislocation, which is usually remedied by relocation and the temporary use of a brace; wear of the metal and plastic joint surfaces, which can contribute to loosening; breakage, which requires a second operation for replacement of the broken component; and damage to nerves or vessels in the area of surgery resulting in temporary or permanent weakness and numbness in the leg.

However, all these complications are rare and state-of-the-art total joint replacement is successful in relieving pain and increasing motion in well over 90 percent of patients undergoing the procedure.

Hospital recovery is usually brief. A continuous passive motion machine may be used on the knee after total knee replacement. Most patients can handle their tasks of living with increased facility and enjoy a more independent mobile lifestyle after total joint replacement. However, the total joint does not have the biologic capacities of normal tissue and usually cannot be subjected to excessive stresses or strains, such as those imposed by active athletics.

The field of total joint replacement is one of the cutting edges of orthopaedic surgery. The continued efforts of orthopaedists and biomechanical engineers to improve techniques and materials have resulted in quantum leaps over the past few years, enabling dramatic improvement in the functional activity of patients with advanced arthritis who undergo such procedures.

15

Boning Up on History

Whited sepulchres, which indeed appear beautiful outward, but are within full of dead men's bones.

Matthew XXI, 13

Let us now travel down a fascinating byway in the study of bone. The investigation of bones unearthed at archaeological digs by those who specialize in the study of ancient disease (paleopathology) has provided clues to our evolution, elucidated our past, and granted engaging insight into our ascent as a species.

The history of mankind is written in the bones that archaeologists and paleontologists have patiently unearthed and analyzed. Unfortunately for these scientists, most bones ultimately decay to the dust to which the Bible warns we all must return. Nonetheless, this recycling plan of nature is altogether good. It has been estimated that the total weight of all the living things that have ever inhabited our earth would just about equal the weight of the planet itself. If our bones did not decompose, we would all be standing shoulder-deep in the skeletal remains of our ancestors!

However, a few bones do indeed survive. For those who have the ability to read them, these have the stories of many lifetimes engraved on their surfaces. Such bones are usually fossilized by a particular and unique chemical composition of the soil, minerals replacing lost organic manner and then crystallizing, thus preserving the original shape of the bone for millions of years. The dating of such fossils can be accomplished through radioactive methods that include the measurement of carbon 14, which exists in all living matter and degenerates to nitrogen 14 over a 50,000 year continuum. State-of-the-art dating technology now uses the decay of potassium into the gas argon, a slower chemical process that enables dating of fossils back for several million years. DNA technology also has been used to link names to human remains. With this method it was established that bones unearthed in Russia in 1991 were those of Czar Nicholas II and that the man buried as Jesse James in April 1882 was indeed the fabled bandit.

Techniques developed for the study of fossils and ancient forms of life, including humans, have been used by forensic experts to identify skeletal remains and help solve crimes. Human bones can be distinguished from their animal counterparts. The time of death can be reasonably well fixed. Sex can be determined by studying particular parts of the skeleton. For example, the pelvic bones or leg bones in men reflect the greater time that boys spend growing during puberty, a period when the legs are growing faster than the spine. The male forearm is longer than the female forearm at birth, and stays that way, whereas women tend to have longer index and ring fingers. Another sexual difference is broader hips in women (Figure 15-1) and broader shoulders in men, both an expression of hormonal influence. Comparing the bones from five prehistoric people from Illinois, Arizona, and Nubia, scientists have determined that infant mortality was lower than in many poor societies today. Mortality peaked at about age 4 and age 25. Apparently, life was most threatened by nutritional stress after weaning, and from combat, childbirth, and hunting in early adulthood.

Occupation can sometimes be established. As Wolff's law tells us, form follows function in bone. The skeleton of a man buried by the eruption of Mount Vesuvius 1,900 years ago was

FIGURE 15-1 The female pelvis (right) shows broader hips and a larger pelvic outlet.

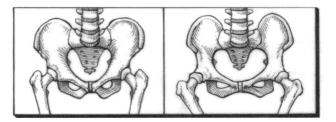

unearthed with his sword by his side. His arm bones were enlarged by years of carrying a shield on the left arm and throwing a javelin with the right (modern rodeo cowboys have similar bony augmentation of the lariat-throwing arm). His knees showed changes from the tension of a horseman's muscles. All of this is evidence of his being part of the Roman professional military, probably the cavalry.

Race can sometimes be ascertained by examining the skull, age is best established by checking dental structure, and height can be estimated by measuring the long bones of the extremities.

One of the most striking changes in ancient skeletons is a general decrease in height after the advent of agriculture.

Disease appears to be as old as life itself. Bacteria (streptococci) have been identified in pre-Cambrian rocks more than 36 million years old. Bony fossils stand in mute testimony to the ravages of prehistoric pathologies. In the Cretaceous era, the period during which the dinosaurs became extinct, changes in their skeletons provide evidence of opisthotonos (spinal rigidity), osteomata (bony tumor), exostoses (bony protuberances), dental caries, arthritis, and osteoperiostitis (inflammation of the covering membrane of bone). Later in the Pliocene period, evidence has been found for the infectious bacterial disease actinomycoses and for spondylitis deformans (a spinal deformation). In the Pleistocene period, the supposed time of transformation of the man-ape into man when paleolithic man roamed Europe, abundant evidence has been discovered of spondylitis deformans, necrosis (bone death), dental caries, exostosis, and osteomyelitis (bony infection).

Even though it is impossible to accurately determine the antiquity of humans or the duration of the various geologic periods, it is unquestioned that disease existed on the earth millions of years before we arrived, and it is becoming increasingly certain that many of the illnesses from which we suffer today also attacked our remote ancestors. Naturally, most of these prehistoric diseases have left evidence of their presence in bones that have resisted the ravages of time. For example, the ape-man or pithecanthropus erectus, who lived approximately one million years ago and whose skeleton was discovered in Java in 1892, revealed a marked exostosis or pathologic bony protuberance of the left thigh bone. This is the earliest record that we have of disease in man.

So-called Harris lines appear in a growing bone after an episode of illness or malnutrition. The distance of this dense line from the end of the bone tells at what age it was laid down. Similar markers called Wilson's bands appear in tooth enamel. Findings such as these indicate disease in ancient populations.

In the later Neolithic (new stone age) period, homo sapiens began to perform the operation of *trephining,* or opening the skull, no doubt employing a flint knife for this purpose. Many such trephined skulls have been unearthed. A particularly fine specimen, preserved in the Berlin Museum of Ethnology, shows an opening equal to one-quarter of the area of the top of the skull. The purpose of these operations is unknown. They may indeed have been performed to treat a depressed skull fracture, or they may simply have been carried out to allow the escape of a "demon" that was causing depression, convulsions, or headache. Neolithic skulls from France also show evidence of local cauterization (burning), which could have been performed for the treatment of epilepsy or melancholia. A number of these specimens reveal bony growth and attempts at repair after the operation, telling us that at least some patients survived this primitive treatment. Well-healed fractures have also been found in many prehistoric skeletons, attesting to the caring attention early humans gave their injured fellows.

Another ancient operation was finger amputation. Pictures on the walls of paleolithic cave dwellers who inhabited France and Spain some 7,000 years ago reveal silhouettes of hands with amputated digits. This practice was widespread as such imprints have also been found in Western parts of the United States, Africa, Australia, Peru, Egypt, Arabia, Israel, Babylonia, Phoenicia, Mexico, and India. Such ritual amputations may have been performed to drive out demons, appease a god, or as a symbol of mourning or even a sign of caste.

Egyptian paleopathology has been particularly fruitful in discovering evidence of disease through the study of mummified bones. Congenital clubfoot, dwarfism, spinal deformity (kyphosis or round-back) secondary to tuberculosis, and bony tumors have all been found.

The farthest reaches of ancient history have been searched by scientists such as Mary and Lewis Leakey and their son Richard. The elder Leakeys devoted their lives to exploring for evidence of ancient man in the Olduvai Gorge, a part of the

African rift valley in the Serengeti plain of Tanzania. There they found specimens of teeth and skull showing that a creature somewhat more evolved than an ape but considerably less than a modern human left the forest, stood upright, and walked the savannah almost one and three-quarter million years ago. This being, somewhere halfway between ape and man, averaged four feet in height and probably weighed less than 100 pounds. More than likely he or she foraged in a group and used tools made of stone, wood, and bone.

A mere decade after the senior Leakeys discovered their "man" (named Zinj), Richard Leakey found yet another skull that pushed the age of mankind back almost another million years while exploring the banks of Kenya's Lake Turkana. Other discoveries by Leakey, particularly the skull known only by its catalog number 1470 in the Kenya National Museum in Nairobi, show clearly that the human brain was enlarging to meet its destiny of dominance in this world.

Almost coincident with Richard Leakey's later finds, Donald Johanssen and his group uncovered the remains of a humanoid female while digging in eastern Ethiopia in 1974. Remarkably, this almost three and one-half million year old skeleton was 40 percent intact. They named her Lucy after the Beatles' song "Lucy in the Sky with Diamonds."

The bones of Neanderthal man, discovered in a limestone cave on a cliff in Germany's Neander valley but subsequently found throughout Europe, indicate that he was bull-necked, had a slouched posture, and was remarkably powerful. Neanderthal man did indeed stand upright and walk with essentially the same posture and gait of a person living today. His brain capacity was about 10 percent greater than that of modern man. There is some evidence that he was a spiritual creature. Not only was he the first to bury his dead, but he cared for the old and infirm. Advanced dating techniques have shown that the Neanderthal man flourished in Europe at least 100,000 years ago. Cro-Magnons, who are anatomically identical to us and from whom we are descended, gradually replaced the Neanderthals over a period of many thousands of years; no trace of the Neanderthals have been found more recently than 35,000 years ago.

Evidence of our physical evolution that would match Darwin's theory of our ascent has been sparse. Pieces to the

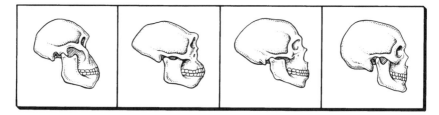

FIGURE 15-2   The Skull from Ape to Man

puzzle were added by Java man, found by the Dutch physician Eugene Dubois in the late 1800s, and Peking man, uncovered in China in the early 1900s. The Piltdown skull, "discovered" by Arthur Smith and Woodward and Charles Dawson in a gravel pit near Piltdown Common, England, though claimed as the "missing link," turned out to be a hoax that matched the skull of a more contemporary human with the jaw of an orangutan (Figure 15-2).

The search continues. It is yet to be ascertained whether the evidence disclosed by ancient bones will tell us that we evolved along the lines of a single species or through several lines that split, allowing extinction of less robust types, or whether early humans coexisted for millions of years, representing separate and distinct lineages. In any case, it is believed that we must look back beyond 5 million years for our common ancestor.

Our past is not so much *cast* in stone, but rather, for those who know how to read its secrets, *etched* in bone.

Epilogue

Some Final Remarks About Better Bones

It has been said that "We see only what we know." This being so, I have tried to help you learn a little more about how you function in health and disease. I have attempted to show you how your skeleton not only supports you physically but also chemically maintains vital aspects of your metabolism. I have shown how important bone is as an archaeological artifact. We have reviewed osteoporosis and arthritis and looked at fractures and fitness. The foot and the hand were discussed, and we talked about bony malformations such as scoliosis as well as tumors and diseases of bone. The common problems of backache and all kinds of shoulder and elbow complaints have been considered. We have examined the neck and the knee. On the way, orthopaedic techniques from arthroscopy to total joint replacement have been covered. Diet and exercise were outlined. You have been given advice on when and how to take care of yourself, and when specifically not to treat yourself but rather to seek expert medical attention.

What, then, does the future hold? Which research possibilities of today could provide therapies for tomorrow? The tools and techniques of molecular biology will provide us with means of entering and correcting defective genes. Genetically determined diseases of bone could then be treated at their source. A gene (Cbfa1) was recently discovered that encodes for a protein that can turn on many other genes normally active in bone formation. Some day doctors may be able to use this gene or its protein to generate new bone in adults, perhaps to treat osteoporosis or allied conditions. Such technology may also change the way we diagnose and manage rheumatic diseases. Continued research in the field of biomedical engineering will no doubt provide metals, plastics, bone cement, and bone glues that are not only biologically compatible when introduced into a living body, but whose physical qualities more closely approximate those of the living tissue they replace.

Bone banking and bone transplant techniques will be further refined to enable even more successful transplantation of human bone and cartilage from donor to recipient, avoiding the potential complications of introducing foreign material into the body. Research is currently being conducted in the development of artificial bone. Several prototypes, including tropical coral, are already in use. The availability of biocompatible artificial bone would obviate the need to use donor bone in those situations where a bone graft is required.

Research into the metabolism of bone proceeds apace. The techniques that bone uses to heal itself are being investigated. From this research, substances that stimulate and control bone growth may be isolated and perhaps even synthesized. These, as well as improved electromagnetic bone stimulators, could be used to treat a variety of injuries and diseases of bone. The pharmaceutical industry is studying new products to inhibit the arthritic process.

Surgical techniques under investigation include cartilage grafting instead of joint replacement. New instrumentation and techniques are being developed to diagnose orthopaedic problems and treat them surgically with minimal operative invasion and trauma. One example of many is the nucleotome technique, with which a herniated lumbar disc can be removed through a small incision. Various new fixation devices are being developed for the treatment of fractures. Some of these are for use inside the body, such as the locked nail used in the treatment of certain fractures of the femur. This device is placed in the medullary canal of the femur and held by screws at each end. This prevents the nail or the bony fragments from rotating. In this way the fracture is rigidly held, and can heal. Internal fixation devices, which absorb after the fracture has healed, are currently in use.

A host of different proteins have been found to induce bone repair by stimulating the expression of immature cells that have the potential to differentiate into osteoblasts. One such protein, produced by recombinant gene technology and called *bone morphogenic protein*, was as effective as bone graft in inducing healing in animal models. On the other hand, smoking has been shown to have an adverse effect on the rate of bone production. In one study, a delay in the average time of healing in closed tibial fractures occurred in smokers (276 days) compared with nonsmokers (146 days).

These are just a few of the many advances that orthopaedic research has already brought us and promises to bring in the future. I emphasize just a few; stick around, there is more to come!

Well, if you have any bones of contention concerning *All About Bone* or the information it offers, I would be pleased to know what they are so I can make proper amends in future editions.

In the meantime, I sincerely hope you have enjoyed reading the book and profited from it as well. The Bible tells us that "God will strengthen my bones. . . ." Indeed He will, but only with your help. So good luck, and stay fit.

Glossary

ABDUCTION: Movement of a part away from the body's center.

ACHILLES TENDON: The largest tendon in the body. It connects the calf muscles to the heel bone.

ACROMION: A bony shelf from the shoulder blade which roofs the shoulder joint. The acromioclavicular (AC) joint connects the acromion to the clavicle.

ADDUCTION: Movement of a body part toward the body's midline or center.

AEROBIC EXERCISE: Exercise utilizing oxygen through deep breathing. Aerobic exercise increases cardiovascular fitness.

ANALGESIC: A pain-relieving drug.

ANTERIOR CRUCIATE LIGAMENT: The crossed ligament inside the knee that lies toward the front (anterior) of the joint. Together with the posterior cruciate ligament, it stabilizes the knee.

ANTERIOR DRAWER TEST: A test for detecting damage to the anterior cruciate ligament.

ARTHRITIS: Damage to a joint. This may be due to inflammation, trauma, infection, degenerative processes, etc.

ARTHROGRAPHY: An x-ray technique utilizing the injection of a contrast dye or air into a joint, allowing its contents to be visualized.

ARTHROSCOPY: A surgical technique for visualizing and operating within a joint (often a knee) which utilizes a fiberoptic light source and a thin tube containing a miniature video system.

BAKER'S CYST: A large sac at the back of the knee, filled with fluid.

BLACK TOENAIL: Bleeding under the nail.

BLISTER: A swelling of the top layer of the skin that occurs due to friction. Blisters contain watery fluid and sometimes blood.

BONY ARCHITECTURE: The microscopic structure of bone that enables it to support body weight.

BONE FORMATION: The secretion and formation of bone matrix by osteoblasts that draws minerals from the blood stream to produce new bone.

BONE MASS: The amount of bone that comprises the skeleton. Bone mass is influenced by nutrition, exercise, and heredity. It reaches its peak at about age 35.

BONE MATRIX: The protein part of bone that gives bone its elastic feature. Bone matrix makes up about half of bone volume but only one-third its weight.

BONE MINERAL: The crystalline part of bone that lends bone its rigid character. Calcium and phosphorus are the principal minerals involved.

BONE REMODELING: A microscopic process of repair of bone in which specialized cells (osteoblasts and osteoclasts) remove old bone, replacing it with new bone.

BONE RESORPTION: The process of bony remodeling in which osteoclasts evacuate old bone, allowing new bone formation to then proceed.

BONE SCAN: The procedure for determining bone mass and mineral density. It is also used to localize and measure uptake and intensity of certain radioactive markers in bone.

BRUISE: Skin discoloration (ecchymosis) produced by ruptured blood vessels beneath the skin, usually caused by a blow. A bruise is sometimes produced by a contusion.

BUNION: Swelling and/or deformity of the joint at the base of the great toe.

BURSA: A moist sac placed where body parts (tendon, muscle, bone, etc.) move against each other. Its purpose is to reduce friction. Bursitis is inflammation of a bursa.

CALCITONIN: A hormone produced by the thyroid gland that acts on osteoclasts to reduce bone resorption.

CALCIUM SUPPLEMENT: Chemical calcium to be taken as a medicine, as distinguished from calcium in the diet.

CALLUS: Thickening of the skin over body parts that are subject to friction or pressure.

CARPAL TUNNEL: A tunnel deep to the palm side of the wrist that contains tendons connecing the muscles of the forearm to the fingers. The median nerve passes through the carpal tunnel.

CARPALS: The eight bones of the wrist.

CARTILAGE: The dense elastic connective tissue that covers the ends of bones at joints. Special cartilage also supports the nose and ears.

CHONDROMALACIA: Degenerative softening of the cartilage in a joint. Chondromalacia patella is due to wear and tear in the kneecap caused by malalignment or overuse.

CHYMOPAPAIN: The active principle of papaya fruit, used in chemonucleolysis, a surgical technique in which chymopapain is injected to dissolve the center of a ruptured disc.

CLAVICLE: Collarbone.

COCCYX: Tailbone.

COLLAGEN: The principal protein of bone, as well as of tendons, skin, ligaments, and cartilage.

COLLATERAL LIGAMENTS: Ligaments running along the side of a joint. In the knee the lateral (outside) collateral ligament and the medial (inside) collateral ligament connect the femur to the tibia and provide stability by preventing the knee from moving sideways.

CONDYLE: An elliptical eminence occurring at the end of a major bone.

CONNECTIVE TISSUE: The supporting framework of the human body. Skin, tendons, ligaments, fascia, bone, and cartilage are all connective tissues. Collagen is the principal protein of connective tissue.

CONTRAST BATHS: Alternating cold and warm baths used to reduce swelling and pain.

CORN: A callus occurring between or on top of the toes. Between the toes it is often called a soft corn.

CORTICAL BONE: Dense bone that makes up the outer walls of bone. The shafts of long bones such as the radius and ulna, humerus, tibia, fibula, and femur are comprised of cortical bone.

CT: Computerized (axial) tomography—A specialized x-ray technique that visualizes sections of the body.

CYST: A fluid-filled sac.

DEBRIDEMENT: Removal of degenerated debris from a joint, a wound, or elsewhere in the body.

DELTOID: The triangular muscle that covers the shoulder and upper arm. The deltoid raises the arm from the body.

DE QUERVAIN'S DISEASE: Tendinitis of the wrist which affects the tendons that connect the muscles of the forearm to the thumb.

DIETARY CALCIUM: Calcium supplied by food.

DISC: The fibrous tissue spacer found between vertebrae.

DISEASE: "Lack of ease"—A condition of pathology in the body.

DISLOCATION: The complete displacement of bones meeting at a joint. If the displacement is only partial, it is called subluxation.

DORSIFLEX: To flex the foot or hand backwards.

DUPUYTREN'S CONTRACTURE: Scarring of the palmar fascia causing contracture, bringing the fingers into the palm.

EFFUSION: Swelling in a joint caused by an accumulation of fluid or blood.

EMG: Electromyography—A technique for visualizing and measuring the electrical activity of muscle.

ENZYME: A specialized protein that acts as a catalyst in metabolic chemical reactions within living organisms.

EPIPHYSIS: A growth center near the end of a bone.

ESTROGEN: The female sex hormone produced principally by the ovaries.

EXTENSION: Straightening a joint.

FASCIA: The tough fibrous covering that encloses muscles. Inflammation of fascia is called fasciitis.

FEMUR: The thigh bone. This is the body's largest bone.

FIBROSITIS: A condition characterized by muscle pain and stiffness.

FIBULA: The thin outer bone of the leg.

FLEXION: Bending a joint.

FRACTURE: Breakage of a bone or cartilage.

GAMEKEEPER'S THUMB: Injury to the ligaments at the base of the thumb, where the web between the thumb and index finger begins.

GANGLION: A fluid-filled cyst originating from a joint or a tendon sheath.

GASTROCNEMIUS: The muscle of the calf that connects to the Achilles tendon (heel cord).

GOUT: A metabolic disease in which an excess of uric acid is present, characterized by acute joint inflammation.

GREATER TROCHANTER: The knob of bone at the upper outer end of the femur.

HAMSTRINGS: Muscles of the back of the thigh.

HEEL SPUR: A bone spike extending forward from the bottom of the heel bone.

HERNIATED DISC: Rupture of a disc between two vertebrae. This often causes compression of the nerve with pain running down the leg (sciatica).

HIP POINTER: A bruise due to a blow on the pelvic bony ridge.

HORMONE: A chemical substance produced by an organ or gland that is carried by the blood to other organs stimulated by that substance.

HUMERAL EPICONDYLE: The lateral humeral epicondyle is the bony bump on the outside of the elbow. This is the location of the irritation causing "tennis elbow." The medial humeral epicondyle lies on the inside of the elbow. This is the location of discomfort in "little league elbow."

HUMERUS: The bone of the upper arm.

HYPER-: Prefix meaning excessive.

HYPO-: Prefix meaning less.

IDIOPATHIC: Without known cause.

INGROWN TOENAIL: A toenail that grows into the fleshy part of the toe. Onychocryptosis is the scientific name.

ISOMETRIC EXERCISE: Exercise that does not involve any movement of a limb or joint.

ITIS: Suffix meaning inflammation.

JOINT: The place where two bones are joined.

JOINT CAPSULE: The fibrous tissue enclosing a joint.

JOINT SPACE: The space enclosed within the joint. Joints can have a synovial lining, which produces synovial fluid.

JUMPER'S KNEE: Tendinitis of the tendon attaching the kneecap to the tibia.

LAMINECTOMY: Spinal surgery involving the removal of bone from the back (lamina) of the spinal column, usually performed as part of the removal of a ruptured disc, spinal tumor, or other impingement on the spinal cord or its nerves.

LIGAMENT: A tough fibrous band connecting bone to bone.

LORDOSIS: The normal front to rear curve of the low back. Sway-back is hyperlordosis.

MALUNION: Literally, bad union in which a fracture is not properly set and unites with the fracture fragments angulated, rotated, severely overlapped and shortened, or otherwise poorly aligned.

MENISCI: Thick cartilage half-rings that cushion the knee, providing shock absorption. The operation of partial or total removal of a meniscus is called a meniscectomy.

MENOPAUSE: Permanent cessation of ovarian function. This occurs naturally when the ovaries stop producing estrogen, often in the early 50s.

METACARPALS: The five hand bones that connect the wrist bones to the finger bones.

METATARSALS: The five foot bones that connect the toes with the top of the foot.

MORBIDITY: Relative incidence of disease.

MORTALITY: Death.

MYOSITIS OSSIFICANS: A condition of bone forming within muscle. This is due to muscular damage secondary to trauma and bleeding.

NAVICULAR: A boat-shaped bone found in both the wrist and the foot. In the wrist it is sometimes called the scaphoid.

NCV: Nerve conduction velocity—Diagnostic technique that measures the conduction of electricity along a nerve. Useful in diagnosing nerve pressure syndromes and other nerve pathology.

NONUNION: Failure of a bone to unite after fracture.

NSAID: *N*on-*S*teroidal *A*nti-*I*nflammatory *D*rug. A drug, not related to cortisone, that suppresses inflammation in the body and relieves pain.

OCCUPATIONAL THERAPY (OT): Therapy directed toward restoring function after disease or injury. Occupational therapy rehabilitates the patient to perform tasks of daily living.

OLECRANON: The end of the ulna that extends behind the elbow joint.

OLECRANON BURSITIS: Inflammation of the elbow bursa over the olecranon.

OPPOSITION: Thumb pinching.

ORTHOPAEDICS: The medical specialty that deals with the diagnosis and treatment of disorders of the musculoskeletal system. This includes bones, joints, ligaments, muscles, tendons, and other related structures.

ORTHOTICS (sing. orthosis): Appliances designed for balancing the foot. Also used as a synonym for brace.

OSGOOD-SCHLATTER'S DISEASE: Tendinitis at the end of the patellar tendon. It appears to be associated with growth plate immaturity at the front end of the tibia. It usually affects vigorous boys between the ages of 10 and 16. It is self-limited.

OSTEOARTHRITIS: The most common form of arthritis. It usually involves weight-bearing joints and is characterized by cartilage destruction and bony overgrowth.

OSTEOBLAST: Bone-producing cell.

OSTEOCHONDRITIS DISSECANS: A condition that causes a piece of bone and its overlying cartilage to degenerate. If the blood supply is entirely lost, it may separate into a joint, often the ankle or knee.

OSTEOCLAST: Cell that removes bone.

OSTEOCYTE: The basic cell within the structure of bone.

OSTEOGENESIS: Bone production.

OSTEOMALACIA: A disease in which bone matrix fails to mineralize. Although produced by many factors, it can be caused by vitamin D deficiency in adults.

OSTEOPOROSIS: Loss of mineral from bone resulting in bony weakening and a predilection for fracture.

OSTEOTOMY: A surgical procedure that involves breaking a bone and resetting it, often performed to more evenly distribute pressure across a joint.

PARATHYROID HORMONE: A hormone that is essential for calcium metabolism. It is produced by the parathyroid glands, which lie next to the thyroid in the front of the neck.

PATELLA: Kneecap.

PELVIS: The bony ring-like structure (also called the pelvic girdle) to which the legs and the spine are attached.

PERIOSTEUM: The dense fibrous tissue that covers the surface of bone and from which circumferential bone growth occurs.

PHALANGES: The bones of the toes and fingers.

PHYSICAL THERAPY: Rehabilitation directed to the prevention of disability and restoration of function following disease or injury. Physical therapy (PT) utilizes physical methods such as exercise, cold, and heat.

PLANTAR FASCIA: The dense fibrous tissue running along the inside of the sole, from the heel to the base of the toes, that maintains the long arch. Inflammation of this structure is called plantar fasciitis.

PLANTAR NEUROMA: A swollen pinched nerve, usually occurring between the third and fourth toes (Morton's neuroma).

PLICAE: Thin membranous walls within the knee. These are developmental left-overs that usually disappear at the end of fetal growth but sometimes remain, causing irritation in the knee.

POLYMYALGIA RHEUMATICA: This condition mostly affects people over 50. It is characterized by shoulder and hip muscle pain and stiffness and a high sedimentation rate of the blood.

POSTERIOR: Toward the back of the body.

PROGNOSIS: Prediction of the outcome or recovery of a disease.

PRONATION: Turning the hands with the palm downward. Pronation also refers to excessive inward rolling of the ankles.

PSEUDARTHROSIS: False joint. When a fracture fails to unite, it can proceed to form a pseudarthrosis.

QUADRICEPS: The large muscle group in the front of the thigh.

RADIUS: The outer bone of the forearm.

REDUCTION: The restoration of a displaced part of the body to its normal position. The "setting" of a fracture involves reduction of the bony fragments to their anatomic pre-fracture position.

RHEUMATOID ARTHRITIS: The second most common form of arthritis. Rheumatoid arthritis is an inflammatory condition of the synovial lining of joints.

RHEUMATOLOGIST: A medical physician who specializes in the diagnosis and treatment of rheumatic diseases.

RICKETS: A childhood disease characterized by defective bone formation with severe deformities of the skeleton. Rickets is most often due to a deficiency of vitamin D.

SACRUM: The lowest fused portion of the backbone.

SCAPULA: Shoulder blade.

SCIATICA: Irritation of the sciatic nerve, the large nerve that supplies motion and sensation to much of the leg from the hip down.

SCOLIOSIS: A side to side curve of the spine.

SEDIMENTATION RATE: A laboratory blood test that can indicate inflammation in the body.

SESAMOID BONES: Tiny bones within tendons that lie under the great toe. Irritation of the sesamoid bones is called sesamoiditis. Strictly speaking, the patella is a sesamoid bone.

SHIN SPLINTS: Pain in the front of the lower leg usually due to increased pressure within the limb secondary to over-exercise.

SNAPPING HIP: Popping at the outside of the hip joint. This is usually caused by a tendon snapping over bone.

SODIUM FLUORIDE: A chemical prescribed to strengthen bone.

SPINAL COLUMN: The flexible bony column that extends from the skull through the low back. It surrounds and protects the spinal cord.

SPINAL FUSION: A surgical operation in which the spine is straightened and kept rigid, often through the use of metallic appliances augmented with bone grafts.

SPINAL STENOSIS: An arthritic condition usually found in older individuals in which the spinal canal is narrowed, causing pressure on the spinal nerves.

SPRAIN: A stretch or tear of a ligament.

STRESS FRACTURE: A hairline fracture caused by stress to the bone. It is often too fine to appear on ordinary x-rays, requiring a bone scan for diagnosis.

STRESS X-RAY: An x-ray taken while a joint is stressed.

SYMPATHETIC DYSTROPHY OR REFLEX SYMPATHETIC DYSTROPHY (RSD): A painful condition characterized by swelling, discoloration, and osteoporosis of a hand or foot, often after a minor injury. Sympathetic dystrophy is due to dysfunction of the sympathetic nervous system. The wasting (atrophy) of bone that occurs in sympathetic dystrophy is called Sudeck's atrophy.

SYNDROME: A collection of signs and symptoms characterizing an abnormal condition.

SYNOVIAL FLUID: The thick colorless lubricating fluid contained within a joint or bursa.

SYNOVIAL MEMBRANE: The joint lining that produces synovial fluid. Inflammation of the synovium is called synovitis.

TALUS: The lowest ankle bone.

TENDON: Fibrous tissue cords attaching muscle to bone. Inflammation of a tendon is called tendinitis.

TENS: *T*ranscutaneous *E*lectrical *N*erve *S*timulation. A technique for pain relief by stimulation of nerves through wires connected to the skin, powered by a small battery carried by the patient.

TERRIBLE TRIAD: A major knee injury involving tearing of the medial meniscus and rupture of both medial collateral and anterior cruciate ligaments.

TIBIA: The larger of the lower leg bones (the shin bone).

TOTAL JOINT REPLACEMENT: Surgery replacing a joint with metal and plastic components. Cemented and non-cemented types are available.

TRABECULAR BONE: The spongy bone that fills the ends of long bones, the central portion of the vertebrae, and the inside of flat bones.

TRACTION: Pull applied to a limb through the use of weights and pulleys.

ULNA: The inner bone of the forearm.

ULTRASOUND: High frequency sound waves used for therapy. Ultrasound produces heat in deep body tissues. Ultrasound can also be used for diagnostic purposes (ultrasonography).

URIC ACID: A waste product of the body. An excess of uric acid can lead to gout.

VERTEBRAE: The small bones making up the spinal column.

VITAMIN D: A substance that increases the capacity to absorb dietary calcium. It is not a true vitamin as it is produced in the human body when the skin is exposed to sunlight.

WEAVER'S BOTTOM: Ischial bursitis.

Index

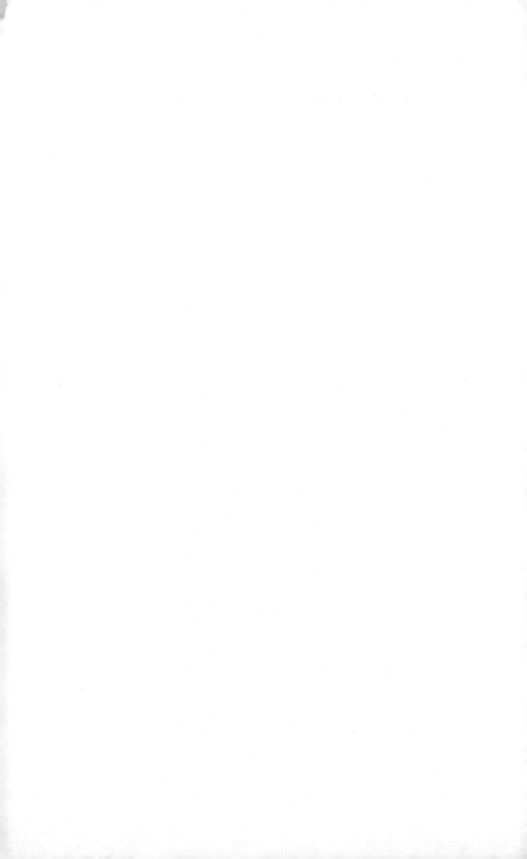